RAISE YOUR WINE I.Q.— AND INCREASE YOUR HEALTH

—What vital group of vitamins is found in a glass of wine?

—How many calories does wine have?

—How can you use wine to improve your complexion?

—What do men and women say about wine and their sex lives?

—What do prominent doctors say about the therapuetic properties of wine?

—What wine is best for the common cold?

—What are the differences among wines, and what differences do they make to you?

These are just a few of the questions answered in the one guide that uncorks all the natural goodness and health-giving benefits of wine for you to sample, savor and enjoy in so many wonderful ways.

STAY HEALTHY WITH WINE

STAY HEALTHY WITH WINE

Natural Cures and Beauty Secrets from the Vineyards

Marjorie Michaels

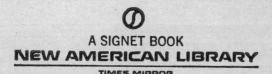

A SIGNET BOOK

NEW AMERICAN LIBRARY

TIMES MIRROR

PUBLISHER'S NOTE

The ideas, procedures, and suggestions contained in this book are not intended as a substitute for consulting with your physician. All matters regarding your health require medical supervision.

Copyright © 1981 by Marjorie Michaels

This is an authorized reprint of a hardcover edition published by The Dial Press.

First Signet Printing, September, 1982

1 2 3 4 5 6 7 8 9

To Pat and Phil,
two of my healthiest friends,
who have given me
understanding and friendship
Prosit.

CONTENTS

Wine is like music.
The more you know about it,
the more you enjoy it.

—Frank Schoonmaker

FOREWORD

Is wine good for what ails you?

In recent years, Americans have become preoccupied with good health. As a direct result of our increased interest in physical fitness, hundreds of books have been written on beauty, diet, and exercise. The entire country has gone jogging-crazy, and gourmet cooking now leans toward the slim-line. America is also going through a wine-drinking revolution. Since 1970, wine consumption has increased sharply relative to that of hard liquor as more and more people ask for a glass of white wine rather than the traditional martini. The time has come to take a serious look at wine, not how or what to buy, but its effects on beauty, health, nutrition, and physical fitness.

Archaeologists believe that grape wine was made as early as ten thousand years ago. Wine was long preferred to water because it was cleaner and safer to drink. Today, our "purified" water is becoming increasingly polluted with chemicals. Recently the quality of our drinking water has caused major medical controversies, and many diseases have been linked directly to our drinking water supplies. Once thought to be the purest of drinks, water can actually contribute to major illness. Kidney stones have been linked to high levels of calcium found in drinking water. Medical research now indicates that people run a higher risk of heart disease when drinking water that has heavy calcium deposits. The asbestos levels of many city water supplies have been proved to be carcinogenic. Based on these findings and many others concerning the chemicals found in our drinking water and their relationship to disease, is it any wonder that more people are rediscovering the good, pure qualities of wine?

Wine has always been associated with the art of good living, inspiration, and creativity, as well as being a welcome symbol of hospitality. How can any man-made chemical concoction compete with nature's own pure drink?

Never before has such interest been shown in international cuisine. Every month gourmet magazines and cookbooks detail the fantastic foods and wines of countries around the world. It would be impossible to think of enjoying a gastronomic feast without the subtle pleasures of a good bottle of wine. "A meal without wine is a day without sunshine," is a popular French proverb. A meal with wine is eaten slowly, as it should be, because wine must be sipped to be thoroughly enjoyed; the bouquet must linger on the palate as the wine begins to spread its beautiful warmth throughout the entire body. You linger, enjoy, you dine. Wine aids digestion, stimulates the gastric juices naturally, as well as bringing out the flavor and savor of food. Wine is the natural complement to food. Good food and good wine are together the perfect combination.

This is a book about wine and its effect on your health, by a wine-lover. In seeking medical and physiological data, I have interviewed hundreds of physicians in the major wine-growing countries of the World. But I did not stop there, because I discovered quickly that the "experts" were not the final word. So I spent over a year interviewing patients who had been treated with wine therapy. Their experiences and suggestions have been invaluable in writing this book.

Medical science today is once again taking a long and serious look at wine and the use of wine therapy. Of course, guidelines must be established, and physicians must be openminded if their patients are interested in substituting wine for the normally prescribed medication. They must be objective, offering specific advice and definite recommendations that will, on both a preventive and a curative program, detail how much and how often people should drink various wines.

When the two basic rules of wine therapy are followed —distinguishing the quality of the wine and consuming the recommended quantities—there is very little possibility that wine can become a damaging drink. Wine therapy does not pretend to replace your family doctor but offers an alternative approach to treatment. In many cases, wine can be naturally substituted for modern chemical medications. I hope the reader will find wine therapy helpful and gradually develop a new feeling of well-being and enjoy a healthier life.

= PART ONE =

WINE AND
YOUR HEALTH

CHAPTER ONE

WINE AND YOUR HEALTH

WINE THERAPY

Wine therapy has been used successfully throughout Europe as well as other regions where wine is commonplace, for centuries. Doctors have developed a fairly standardized wine therapy for specific health problems. In addition, many medical researchers feel strongly that wine, when taken on a regular basis, can play a definite role in preventing certain illnesses. Physicians throughout the United States have gradually begun, during the last few years, to prescribe wine therapy to their patients with more conviction as knowledge of the therapeutic uses of wine becomes more widespread.

For many years California had an official agency, the Wine Advisory Board, that authorized research into the medical aspects of wine. Dr. Milton Silverman, former head of medical research for the Board, and a world-famous pharmacologist and wine writer, states, "Because of its low alcohol content and its content of protective chemicals, and also because of cultural and sociological factors . . . wine may . . . be described as a pharmaceutical agent of major importance, and moreover, an agent which may serve as the most effective preventative of alcoholism known to medicine. Beyond a certain point, wine and plain alcohol differ. More wine continues to give more relief, while plain alcohol or more of a comparable beverage begins to give more tension."

In the following chapters you will find the most up-to-date conclusions dealing with wine and health. Wine has many positive attributes, but is not a cure-all. In many cases, how-

3

ever, wine can play a direct curative role. It can also aid many other therapeutic medications by adding to their over-all effectiveness. The excessive use of wine to the point of al-coholism is very rare. When wine is used as a food in conjunction with other foods at mealtimes, it can play an im-portant role in developing social and cultural protective pat-terns against alcoholism.

Wine is a natural and mild tranquilizer that can help com-bat emotional tensions and anxieties without causing depen-dence. Relaxation is an important part of our entire health cycle. Unfortunately, more and more Americans find them-selves unable to cope with the tensions of modern life, and turn to the artifice of chemical relaxants and tranquilizers for relief. Many of these drugs can cause unpleasant side ef-fects, ranging from slight drowsiness, dizziness, nausea, vomit-ing, and tremors, to serious epileptiform seizures. Many tranquilizers cause mental depression that can seriously affect your psychological well-being.

Wine, on the other hand, enhances your life. If a medica-tion is to be wholly successful, it should produce a positive psychological effect as well as a physical one. At bedtime, if given the choice of a little yellow pill—which could cause a serious side effect—or a two- to four-ounce glass of a deli-cious dessert wine that has been used for years as a mild and safe sedative, which would you choose? When given a choice between prescribing a tranquilizer or wine, most doc-tors prefer a pill. Why? Perhaps because it's much easier!

The safety of wine is known, whereas new side reactions to tranquilizers are being discovered daily. Why should our medical profession ignore the positive qualities of wine, one of the gentlest tranquilizers known that is free from side ef-fects?

During the past decade medicine has changed its perspec-tive from curative to preventive. In this respect, wine can play an important role in the daily diet. Nutritionally, when used in the normal diet, wine provides energy and aids in di-gestion. Recent medical research programs suggest that wine, when used in the daily diet, may act as a protective factor against coronary disease. Wine can help prevent recurrent at-tacks of angina pectoris, which are caused by spasms of the blood vessels within the heart.

Not only convalescent facilities, but hospitals in thirty-five states now offer the service of wine to patients. The program

4

is designed to make the patients' stay in the hospital more relaxing and enjoyable. Surveys of these programs show that wine, when served with the evening meal, increases the patients' satisfaction, aids digestion, and helps most to sleep better.

Wine has always been widely prescribed by physicians in European hospitals. While researching this book, I uncovered some very interesting data concerning wine consumption in the Elisabeth Hospital in Darmstadt, Germany. In 1871 during a six-month period, 755 patients were treated with 4,633 bottles of white wine, 6,233 bottles of red wine, 60 bottles of Champagne, and 350 bottles of port wine!

Wine is an intriguing food that supplies a substantial part of the body's energy requirements. Many doctors are incorporating dry wines into reducing diets. Case studies show that when this approach is taken, most dieters decrease their carbohydrate intake. Dry wine, with only about twenty-four calories per ounce, taken in moderation, will never unbalance a diet.

The Society of Medical Friends of Wine was established almost forty years ago in San Francisco to help study the importance of wine, and today its membership consists of several hundred physicians and research specialists. The Society holds regular meetings to evaluate scientific papers concerning the medical and social aspects of wine.

WINE AS AN ANTIBIOTIC

Most evidence of the antibacterial effects of wine has been collected during wartime. Armies, even in early Roman times, used wine to purify drinking water. Wine was also used as an antiseptic for wounds. Recent studies show that phenolic compounds, including the pigments of wine, are important active antibacterial agents. These compounds are extremely effective against the various strains of bacteria responsible for gastrointestinal diseases. The prophylactic effect of wine on intestinal diseases was known by Julius Caesar, who ordered his soldiers to drink red wine every day to prevent illness. French soldiers during Napoleon's reign were issued three and a half liters of wine per day, and the Spanish always stocked their ships with twice as much wine as water.

The antibiotic effect of wine resembles most closely that of penicillin. At the Bonn Institute, in West Germany, the antibacterial action of wine and penicillin were compared, and it was shown that within a fifteen-minute period, a combination of water and wine was substantially more potent against colonies of specific bacteria than strong concentrations of penicillin. The penicillin in the short period of time was unable to act as effectively as the wine. When the experiment was extended over a twenty-four-hour period, the wine was unable to sustain the long-range effect of the penicillin. When the wine was combined with the antibiotic therapy, it increased the overall bacterial action. The wine exerted its immediate destructive action while the antibiotics acted as long-range reinforcements.

Recent research reveals that patients who are taking penicillin or streptomycin may safely drink white wine. Wine does not lower the concentration of these antibiotics in the bloodstream. Patients taking either Aureomycin or Terramycin will benefit by drinking white wine simultaneously with their medication, because the white wine increases and prolongs the level of these two antibiotics in the blood. In addition, the wine acts to alleviate some of the unpleasant side effects, such as nausea, associated with antibiotic therapy.

WINE AS A MEDICATION

The antibacterial properties of wine have been known to the medical and research communities for years. However, two Canadian scientists have recently completed laboratory studies that show red wine is effective in inactivating a variety of harmful viruses as well.

Certain acidic compounds called naturally polymerized phenols, found in the skins of grapes, have proved effective in fighting disease-causing viruses. Research scientists Jack Konowalchuk and Joan I. Speirs, in a report published in 1976 by the *Journal of Applied and Environmental Microbiology*, concluded that all the wines they tested were antiviral. Red wines were found to be more potent than white, most likely because they are fermented with the grape skins, unlike white wines.

Their Ottawa laboratory produced several strains of virus, including those affecting the intestines, stomach, and skin, and causing membrane blisters and polio. The study made no statement concerning the disease-curing properties of wine in humans, as all tests were conducted in a controlled test-tube atmosphere. The positive results are nevertheless encouraging.

Although wine may help many people in various ways, there are certain cases where it should either not be used or used with caution. Wine should never be given to a person with an uncontrollable drinking problem, or used in patients with peptic ulcers, or inflammations of the stomach, throat, mouth, or esophagus. Abstinence should also be observed with acute kidney infections, genitourinary conditions, or disorders of the prostate gland. Doctors seldom suggest wine in cases of stomach cancer or epilepsy. Wine or alcohol in any form can cause adverse reactions with drugs such as chemical tranquilizers, barbiturates, narcotic agents, and a wide range of drugs used for pathological mental conditions, for example Thorazine. Your doctor should always be consulted before you change your normal regimen with the addition of wine.

CHAPTER TWO

THE HEALING POWER OF WINE THROUGH THE CENTURIES

THE MAGIC BEVERAGE

Our ancestors were enlightened drinkers who knew that wine was one of the finest gifts of nature, a natural medicine from the gods. Homer mentions the famous vineyards of ancient Greece to which man owes his health. Ancient doctors had to rely solely on the self-healing properties of nature, prescribing herbal extracts and plant juices to cure as well as to protect their health. Wine acted as a universal medium in which medicinal plants and herbs could be easily dissolved.

The healing powers of wine are a major feature of mythology. For centuries, wine had its own private god, Dionysus, and enjoyed a sacred reputation. Early Egyptian tomb decorations depict viticulture, the harvest, and curative uses of wine. Writing tablets uncovered in Carthage, Tunis, and Morocco supply similar information detailing secret wine cures.

The Greek pharmacologist Dioskurides in his five-volume medical work, *Materice Medica*, written in the first century, A.D., describes in detail the healing properties of wine. He states, "White wine is easy to digest and good for the stomach and digestive tract, while sweet wine is full, heavy, and often upsets the stomach but is good for the bladder and kidneys. The acid of wine aids digestion, stops diarrhea, and acts as a good diuretic. All wine is astringent, slows the pulse, rids the body of poisons. In general, wine is warming, easily digested, improves the appetite, helps you sleep, and gives you 'life-giving properties.' " Most modern physicians agree that Dioskurides' "life-giving properties" refer to the vitamin and mineral content of wine.

For relief of sore throats, Dioskurides recommends mixing grape skins, finely ground flour, and an egg together in a pan, cooking with honey until well mixed, followed by an addition of red wine. This mixture was to be drunk three times daily. Cancerous skin ulcers were treated with warm wine poultices. Up until the early twentieth century, many of Dioskurides' remedies were still being used extensively in Europe and the Orient.

Hippocrates called the wine the universal medicine and detailed his exact observations, descriptions, and cures. He recommended wine for treating wounds, reducing fevers, adding strength during convalescence, curing headaches and diseases of the digestive tract. His papers discuss in detail the effects of specific wines on bodily organs and functions. For more than a thousand years, Hippocrates' papers and observations provided a standard reference for doctors in many countries, with each successive generation benefiting from the past as the science of wine therapy expanded.

Four thousand years ago in China, the Emperor Yu is credited with having discovered the healing properties of wine. After an eight-year war accompanied by disastrous floods and plagues, the emperor worried so much that he could no longer eat or sleep. The doctors despaired until a maid in the palace, Yi Tieh, served him some wine she had made. After tasting the wine, his appetite returned and after several more cups, his worries vanished and he was able to sleep.

In ancient Persia (present-day Iran), which many historians credit as the birthplace of wine, the King Dschemschid noted the healing properties of wine almost two thousand years before Christ. He commanded that the juice of grapes be pressed and brought to him. He set the juice on the touchstone to be blessed and drank daily until the juice became bitter. He decided that the juice had been poisoned and put it aside. Later that day, one of the king's personal slaves became very ill and thought he was going to die, so he decided to poison himself with the "bitter grape juice." Even after drinking only a little, he felt better; he drank more and fell asleep for a day and a night and woke up cured. The king heard the story, drank some of the wine himself and ordered everyone else to do the same. Many sick people regained their health and the wine was given the name "King's Medicine."

An old Arabic quotation states, "The wine skin is a kingdom to him who possesses it, and the kingdom therein, though small, how great it is!"

In Palestine, wine played an increasingly important role beginning in the second millennium B.C. The Old Testament has more than five hundred mentions of the importance of viticulture and wine's healing properties, but it wasn't until the Last Supper that wine attained its highest praise, as Jesus made bread and wine symbols of Christian belief.

Romans were heavy drinkers and spread viticulture throughout the world in the wake of their armies, up the banks of the Rhone, to Lyons, into Burgundy, and up the Rhine. Viticulture flourished well into the Middle Ages when many of the vineyards were taken over by monasteries and the nobility. The monks of this period were master physicians and perfected many medicines based on wine cures. The vineyards of today still correspond very closely to those of the Renaissance, but during the nineteenth century, wine-making methods were greatly improved and closely linked with standard medical practices.

Alcohol was a routine embellishment of American colonial life. The Puritans stocked the Mayflower with what they called "the good creative of God." At the first Thanksgiving, cups were raised with locally fermented wine. Our inventive ancestors, when faced with failing grapes, produced the necessary beverage from artichokes, pumpkins, cornstalks, turnips, and horseradish. "Oh we can make liquor to sweeten our lips of pumpkins, of persnips, of walnut-tree chips," went one early New England ditty.

One famous American, Thomas Jefferson, wrote to President James Monroe in 1817, when he was seventy-six, concerning the state of his health: "Like my friend, Dr. Benjamin Rush, I have lived temperately, eating little animal food. I double, however, the doctor's daily glass-and-a-half of wine, and even treble it with a friend . . ."

In the colonies, many strong white wines were imported from southern Europe and were classified as "sack." In 1646, Governor Winthrop of the Massachusetts Bay Colony mentions the arrival of eight hundred butts of sack in Boston harbor onboard four ships.

The sack posset was an early colonial cure for the cold. The following recipe appeared in the *Practical Housewife* as late as 1860:

Put a quart of raw milk into a saucepan and place it over a slow clear fire. When it boils, crumble four Damascus biscuits into it; give it one boil, remove from the fire, add grated nutmeg and sugar to taste, stir in half a pint of sack and serve.

A very interesting book, and bible of many early Americans, was Samuel Stearns's *The American Herbal*, published in 1801, which contained numerous medicinal alcoholic—and especially wine—remedies to alleviate many illnesses:

Wine: Wines are considered as cordials.
Red port is the most astringent.
Plenish wine is detergent and laxative.
Canary is nutritious and the Spanish white wine is strengthening.
Wine is a stimulant, sedative, expectorant, diaphoretic, inspissant, antalkaline, and antiseptic.
Good wine stimulates the stomach, cheers the spirits, warms the habit, promotes perspiration, renders the vessels full and turgid, raises the pulse, and quickens the circulation.
Claret, Madeira, and port are often used with great success in fevers of a typhus kind, when the stomach is weak, rejects all food, and the wine agrees with the patient. It is good in languors, debilities, the low stage of fevers, and for resisting putrefactors, for those who are aged, weak, relaxed, and exposed to contagion, and a warm, moist corrupted air.

A standard colonial remedy for rheumatism as well as fevers was to pulverize an ounce of prickly ash bark in a pint of a strong red wine or wine brandy.

Wine brandy was a popular American drink consumed for both social and medicinal purposes. Samuel Sterns wrote:

> Brandy is a spirituous inflammable liquor, obtained from wine, and some other liquors by distillation. Wine brandy, made in France, is esteemed the best in Europe, both for drinking and for medicinal purposes. This kind of brandy, drunk with moderation, well diluted with water, strengthens the tone of the nervous system, raises the spirits, and braces the fibres; it is good in the gout, and a variety of other complaints.

It was not until after World War I, with the establishment of Prohibition, that wine came into official disfavor. Physicians, during the period from 1920 to 1933, completely ignored the use of wine in modern medical practice. Coinciding with the repeal of Prohibition, the United States experienced the birth of modern pharmaceutical medicine. Doctors were beginning to demand proof that the new therapeutic substances were more effective than previous remedies. Wine during this period was closely scrutinized for effectiveness, but despite positive natural results, lost out to the newer modern wonder drugs. It has only been recently that Americans have begun to look for natural cures that can in some way replace or complement the chemicals that have so long monopolized medical treatment.

CHAPTER THREE

NATURE'S PERFECT HEALTH FOOD

Before we begin to learn about specific wines' effects on the body, it is important to understand fully what wine is, and how it is made.

Basically, wine is fermented juice from freshly gathered grapes. The actual chemical composition of wine varies, depending on the grape species, soil type, climate, and method of cultivation, as well as the condition of the grapes at harvest. Equally important differences in wines are determined by the type and degree of fermentation.

HOW WINE IS MADE

There are three main phases in wine production: cultivation, gathering and fermentation, and bottling. The vineyard owner never rests, because as soon as this year's vintage (harvest) is over, next year's cultivation must begin. Vines must be grafted, pruned, restaked, and fertilized. In the spring and early summer, the soil must be hoed and weeded so that the topsoil is light and absorbent. This is a very important protective step against later droughts. The vines are sulphured and sprayed to help fight off blight.

A perfect harvest is a rare thing, because so much can happen before the grapes have a chance to ripen. In many small vineyards around the world, the grapes are the vineyard owner's life. He is at the mercy of the weather for the grapes to ripen, rich in grape sugar, ready for a perfect harvest.

BREAKDOWN OF GRAPES AND GRAPE PRODUCTS

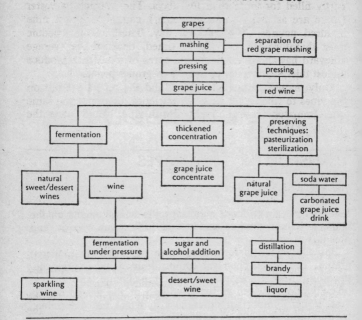

THE HARVEST

Historically the harvest takes place one hundred days after the vines are in full flower. As harvest time approaches, sometime in September or October, depending on whether the summer was sunny and hot or cool and rainy, the vineyard experts pick grapes every two or three days, analyzing the degree of maturity. Charts are made detailing the increase of sugar and decrease of acid content. In timing a harvest, the major factor is the sugar content of the grape. To the uneducated eye, the grape may look ripe, but during the last few days of maturation, grapes synthesize sugar at a daily increase of more than three ounces per gallon of juice. The wait is always a calculated risk, especially if it is a late harvest with the dangers of autumn rains and hailstorms.

Harvesting is very hard work. Only local workers and family members can usually stand the strain. For example, in France a vat in Beaujolais holds approximately sixteen thousand pounds of grapes. Once a vat is started, it cannot be left partly filled for more than two days. The average harvester (there are as many women as men) can pick almost nine hundred pounds of grapes per day. The picking schedule must therefore be very tightly timed, because the average vineyard has about seven to nine acres of vines that produce almost thirty-five thousand pounds of grapes per harvest.

Only mature grapes are picked, and the others are left on the vines to ripen. Not all grape varieties mature at the same rate. Immature grapes, if mixed with ripe, would lower the quality of the wine.

TRANSPORTING THE GRAPES

Harvesting is only the first step. Next the grapes must be removed from the vineyard. Throughout Europe, where most vineyards are steep and narrowly planted, everything must still be done by hand. Containers are usually made from wicker or wood and, although picturesque, are very heavy and uncomfortable to carry when full. In recent years, both plastic and aluminum baskets have begun to replace the wicker back basket, which dates to medieval times.

The containers cannot be too heavily loaded, because the volume of grapes will begin to press before they reach the vats and premature fermentation can take place. This is why iron buckets are never used; even trace amounts of iron in the must (the mixture of grape juice, pulps, seeds, and skins) will create a chemical imbalance, which will ruin the wine.

MAKING THE WINE

When the grapes have finally reached the place where the wine is to be made, sometimes the stalks are removed before pressing. The operation is usually done by a mechanical sieve. In other cases, the stalks are left on to add more body to the wine.

The method of this first pressing or smashing of the grapes varies from area to area, but the reason for the procedure remains the same: to release the grape juice from the skins and allow natural yeasts that live on the grape skins while they are growing to get to the grape sugar in the juice and ferment it. This yeast, called *Saccharomyces*, turns the grapes into wine by converting their natural sugars into ethyl alcohol and carbon dioxide.

FERMENTATION

Wine production is more than just gathering the grapes, pressing, and allowing them to ferment. The fermentation process must be monitored carefully. It is the fermentation that produces the alcohol in wine from the sugar in grapes.

Fermentation is a chemical process in which grape sugars (dextrose and fructose) are transformed into ethyl alcohol and carbon dioxide gas. During the process, the gas is dispersed into the air, leaving the alcohol. The conversion of milk into cheese is a similar process.

Natural yeast, a self-reproducing plant organism, causes fermentation to take place. There are many varieties of yeast, but the one that transforms grape juice into wine is called *Saccharomyces*.

Microscopic *Saccharomyces* spores attach themselves to the grape skins as they ripen. After the grapes are harvested and the juice pressed, the yeast produces enzymes that cause the grape juice to ferment and turn into wine. In the unfermented grape juice the yeasts find the perfect atmosphere to multiply at an astounding rate. This initial yeast growth is made possible by the presence of oxygen in the air, but *Saccharomyces* will not produce alcohol if allowed to continue to grow in an oxygen-rich atmosphere.

Saccharomyces start out working quite violently, but the action subsides as the proportion of sugar is reduced through conversion into alcohol and carbon dioxide. The yeast works best between 65 and 80 degrees F, so the winemaker must control the temperature carefully during fermentation. When the alcohol level reaches about 14 percent, or all the sugar has been used up, the action of the yeast is inhibited and the fermentation process ends.

RACKING

At its peak, though, the wine is far from finished. Racking, the next step, separates the wine from the remaining solid matter that is still in the vats.

This part of the operation involves a second more refined pressing. The first wine out of the press, the dripping wine, *vin de goutte*, is superb. Everyone gathers around for a taste before the harsher *vin de presse* is released. The young wine is then pumped into a cask. Many wine-producing areas still mature the wine in old oak casks. In Germany, a Mosel cask holds up to 264 gallons, while small versions are used along the Rhine (153 gallons), and in Bordeaux (57 gallons) and Burgundy (58 gallons). In the California area, where oak is expensive, casks are made from redwood to hold 160 gallons.

Not all vineyards age their wine by the traditional cask method. In many areas, glass-lined cement vats or stainless-steel tanks are being utilized. These large-volume cement vats are ideal for producing wines that are fruity and can be drunk relatively young. Wooden vats are still necessary if the wine requires slow oxidation to develop a unique bouquet.

MATURING

In the first few months in the cask, the wine becomes more refined and the taste is less acid. It is now the winemaker's job to insure that the wine is kept stable. There are no set rules or formulas for this important step, but constant care and tasting is important because each vintage is individual.

BOTTLING

There is no standard time for this operation.

Each wine type is bottled at different times of the year. If a wine is bottled too early a second, different type of fermentation can begin in the bottle, which, among other things, may cause excessive deposits of mineral salts; bottled too late, the wine can lose freshness of taste. White wines are usually bottled from six to eight months after harvesting. Fruitier red wines must be bottled early to retain their fresh taste, while wines from the Médoc or Bordeaux area remain in the casks for up to two years, sometimes more.

No wine should be drunk right after it is bottled, as the taste suffers from the procedure. A wine should rest for one to two months as it begins to age.

WHITE WINES

Different methods are used to make wines, depending upon whether you are making white, red, or rosé wines.

The major difference between white and red wine is that white is made by fermenting the freshly pressed juice only. There is no maceration with the skins, although a certain amount of leaching is expected during crushing or pressing.

White wine production must be rapid to insure limited contact of the crushed grapes with air and make sure that the fermenting must does not extract tannin and coloring matter from the solid parts that come in contact with the juice. It takes approximately six to twelve hours for the solid matter to settle, while the clear juice is drawn off for fermentation. To insure that fermentation does not begin too soon, small amounts of sulphur dioxide are put into the clearing vats where the must waits to be pumped off.

In sweet white wine production, fermentation must be interrupted before all the sugar has been converted. This can occur naturally if the alcohol content becomes too high for the yeasts to live, or the winemaker may add sulphur.

RED WINES

Red wine production is more complex. Time plays an important role, and fermentation can take anywhere from three days to three weeks. The shorter the fermentation time, the less time required to mature. It is also an art to determine how long the juice is allowed contact with the solid matter. This varies from wine to wine. The length of time it remains in the vat can determine the acidity . . . too high after a cold summer, too low after a hot summer.

Many vineyards are experimenting with yeasts on the theory that a particular yeast will give the finished wine a specific characteristic. Beaujolais and Chambertin yeasts as well as many other yeasts are available. Yeasts are important not only for turning sugar into alcohol, but also for the many substances they produce that help shape the wine's final character.

ROSÉ WINES

A true rosé is not a mixture of red and white wines, but a wine in which the grape skins are allowed to remain in the vat after crushing long enough to tint the wine pink. Up until the eighteenth century, rosé wines were popular, but lost favor until after World War I.

Rosé wine is a contradiction, combining two objectives that are in opposition: to achieve the best color, but also to make the wine as light, delicate, and elegant as possible. The beginning of the rosé-making process is like that for red wine, but the end is rapid, like that for white. Only juice from the first pressing is used to make rosé wine, because the second and third pressings are too deeply colored and are usually added to red wine vats.

Sulphur is usually added to retard fermentation for the first twenty-four to forty-eight hours. During this time the solid material settles and can be removed. Then fermentation can begin. This is the normal procedure for most Burgundy, Anjou, and Touraine rosés.

Most rosé wines are bottled early to preserve their fruitiness.

A CHEMICAL BREAKDOWN OF WINE

A chemical breakdown of a dry table wine reveals a solution composed of approximately 85 percent water, 12 percent ethyl alcohol, and 3 percent various mineral and vegetable substances. Despite the small proportion of the latter compounds, combined they have the greatest effect on the eventual quality of the wine.

During a wet vintage, because most of the *Saccharomyces* have been washed off by the heavy rainfall, fermentation is slower and will produce an unsatisfactory wine. Not only is the condition of the grapes at harvest significant, but a regulated temperature to encourage the immediate growth of the *Saccharomyces* is of vital importance.

But wine is not just grape juice with its sugars changed into alcohol and carbon dioxide. Minute quantities of other substances are present and may be divided into two main categories: those present in the original grape juice that have not been altered by fermentation, and those that are by-products of the fermentation. Grape sugar, various acids, *Saccharomyces*, cellulose, and essential oils fall into the first category. Glycerine, various acids, alcohols other than ethyl, as well as volatile esters and aldehydes fall into the second. Esters, organic compounds responsible for the fruity bouquet, are formed during maturation by the combination of various acids and the alcohol in the wine. Aldehydes, organic compounds that affect the color and flavor of wine, increase gradually during fermentation.

Butyl, propyl, and amyl alcohols are found in minute quantities in most normal wines and, like all alcohols, have the ability to form various esters and acids which play an important role in forming the wine's bouquet or aroma. The excellence of the wine is determined by the various acids—succinic, acetic, propionic, and valerianic—that appear in the wine in very small quantities. These acids do not alter the taste of the wine, but are responsible for the bouquet, the savor.

The amount of grape sugar that remains in the wine after fermentation depends on two facts: the amount of grape sugar in the original juice, and the type of fermentation. In fortified or "sweet" wines, the sweeter the original grape juice, the sweeter the wine; port, for example, relies on the addition of brandy during fermentation. Sauternes use rich, overripe grapes. This rule does not apply to beverage wines where the reverse is often the case. The greater the amount of sugar in the grape juice, the higher the alcohol content of the wine.

Saccharomyces are extremely fine and light particles. They remain suspended in the must until the end of the fermentation process. Some attach themselves to microscopic particles of cream of tartar and settle to the bottom of the vats. Others combine chemically with other substances, and still others remain intact in the finished wine.

Cream of tartar is formed by the principal acid in the grape juice, tartaric acid. Because cream of tartar is soluble in water but not in alcohol at cool temperatures, it forms small white crystals in wine. The particles are heavier than wine and settle to the bottom of the bottle. Cream of tartar plays an important role in the bottle. If the wine is stored correctly in a cool cellar, the cream of tartar will crystalize, clinging to the sides of the bottle, and eventually falling to the bottom. The precipitation is desirable because it helps remove any extra acidity, making the wine "smoother" to the taste.

The natural acidity of the grape juice is of enormous benefit in the wine-making process because it stops bacterial development and aids the normal growth of the yeasts. The acid found in the greatest concentration in wine is acetic acid. The formation of this acid is in direct proportion to the amount of alcohol in the wine and the amount of oxygen present: a wine with a high alcoholic content that has very little exposure to oxygen will form a small quantity of acetic acid. If wine with a low alcoholic level is kept in a fairly warm place and exposed to air, its alcohol will soon become acetic acid. If a vinegary taste is detected, the wine has turned as a result of air reaching the wine. This usually occurs if the wine has been improperly stored or a poor cork has been used. It is important that wine bottles be properly stored lying down so that the cork stays wet and does not dry out and shrink.

But acetic acid is not all bad, because it plays an important part in developing the flavor and bouquet of the wine by dissolving various mineral salts.

Another important element found in wine is glycerine. One liter of wine contains from about five to fifteen grams of glycerine, which is in part responsible for the wine's individual character, producing what connoisseurs call "body."

Generally, the higher the alcoholic content, the less bouquet a wine has. Most of the heavy wines of southern Europe have little or no bouquet, while many of the wines of northern Europe have rich, fragrant bouquets. The alcoholic content of American wines varies more with respect to the producer than by region.

Wine is defined by weight in terms of alcoholic content as follows:

	Grams of alcohol per liter
Country wines	50–70 grams
Table wines	60–80 grams
Heavy wines	100 grams

STATED IN PERCENTAGES, THE ALCOHOLIC CONTENT OF VARIOUS WINES IS:

Mosel/light white wines	8–9%
Some French red wines/most table wines	8–10%
Heavier or fortified wines	12% or more

If the heaviness of the wine comes from the alcohol content, the fresh lightness comes from the acid content. The rich, interesting, spicy taste of some wines lies on the delicate border between the alcohol and acid balance.

If a wine is well-balanced, there will be a ratio of 10 percent alcohol to 1 percent acid. In general, one liter of wine contains from five to ten grams of acid. In general red wines have a lower acid content than white wines. Most wines reach their peak in seven to ten years, but many local table wines that do not have proper acid balances have very short lives and must be drunk almost immediately. Doctors say that in southern Europe, where most of the wine is rich in alcohol and poor in acids, lemon juice is often added to preserve it, frequently causing acute acid indigestion.

Sulphuric acid is added to prevent post-fermentation oxidation, or "hold" sweetness in cheap wines, but when too much is present, the wine tastes hard and flat. Sulphiting is common practice in most modern wineries. In Common Market countries, the amount of sulphuric acid that may be added is limited to 175–400 mg. per liter, but in many other countries around the world where the laws are more liberal, greater amounts may be present, which can produce severe headaches and stomach pains. Many cheap Liebfraumilchs and white Bordeauxs reek of sulphur.

MINERAL CONTENT OF WINE

The mineral content of wine is determined by the amount of yeast available during fermentation. People can assimilate minerals only in conjunction with either plant or animal substances such as organic salts. The mineral salts present in wine are all ready to be assimilated in their ionized form. In red wine phosphorus is found in the form of phosphate. The concentration of a mineral can vary according to the wine from a trace to more than 50 percent of the minimum daily requirement.

PHOSPHORUS

Phosphorus, in alliance with calcium, is necessary for healthy bone tissue and plays a simple but important role in maintaining the acid balance of the blood. It accelerates the nitrogen exchange of the metabolism and has an important influence on the fat and sugar balance in the body, which is essential for the free exchange of energy needed for muscle contractions.

SULPHUR

Sulphur, in the form of sulphate, is found in practically all types of wine. This is especially important for the protection of the liver, which functions as a protective filter against harmful microorganisms and organic poisons.

FLUORIDE

Fluoride, also found in wine, plays an important part in preserving the soft tissues of the body.

CALCIUM

Wine is naturally high in calcium, the most abundant mineral found in the body. It is deposited almost entirely (99 percent) in the bones and teeth, and a small amount is present in the soft tissues. In order for calcium to function properly, adequate amounts of phosphorus, magnesium, and the vitamins A, C, and D are necessary. Calcium is poorly absorbed by the body, which utilizes only about 30 percent of the actual amount ingested. And yet calcium is important for good health. The body requires it for proper blood clotting, heart regulation, normal nerve transmission, and muscle functioning.

Deficiencies produce a wide variety of symptoms which include nervousness, excessive menstruation, leg cramps, stunted growth, poor bone and teeth formation, dry hair, brittle nails, and eczema.

IRON

Iron deficiencies are very common, affecting an estimated 25 percent of the U.S. population. Iron deficiencies produce anemia, which is associated with abnormal fatigue and pale skin, loss of appetite, and shortness of breath.

Wine is an *excellent* source of iron. Forty percent of the body's daily iron requirement is contained in one-half liter of wine. The normal daily requirement for iron is approximately 5.5 mg. Port wine is exceptionally high in iron content—3.5 mg. per liter—and has been used for years for treating iron-deficiency anemia. Sherry, Bordeaux and Burgundy wines also have high iron concentrations.

POTASSIUM

The average daily requirement of potassium is approximately 2500 mg., which is twice the amount required of phosphorus or calcium. Potassium is important for healthy nerve cells that control muscle contractions, as a stimulant for the kidneys, and combines with sodium to regulate fluids. Wine is an excellent source of potassium, with an average of 800 mg. per liter.

Deficiencies cause nervousness, muscular weakness, edema, and tachycardia, or irregular heartbeat. The majority of potassium deficiencies follow vomiting, diarrhea, or the use of diuretics.

SODIUM

The primary function of sodium is to work with chlorine to regulate the acidity of the body fluids. The balance between the two must be maintained if the kidneys are to operate properly by excreting chlorine when the body's acid balance is acid and sodium when it is alkaline.

Sodium deficiencies cause dehydration, weakness, fainting, and mental confusion, but an excess can lead to edema, hypertension, and eventual renal damage.

The average American diet is very high in sodium, especially artificially softened water. Most wines are extremely low in sodium—less than 100 mg. per liter—and provide an excellent dietary supplement, especially for high blood pressure sufferers who must regulate their sodium intake.

WINE AND VITAMINS

Wine contains at least ten vitamins in significant amounts, especially the B vitamins, including thiamine and riboflavin. Of the ten "growth factors" needed for human well-being, more than half are present in wine. All of these vitamins are natural, not synthetic as much of our food and vitamins have become today. Wine vitamins are produced from living organisms, and therefore we must begin to think of wine also in these terms, as a living, natural drink.

When vitamins are supplied in natural form it is easier for the body to assimilate them. As the body is able to store very few vitamins, vitamins must be regularly supplied. Wine is rich in natural vitamins.

Recent studies have shown that small quantities of the essential B-complex vitamins are found in wine. They include B_1, riboflavin, pyridoxine, pantothenic acid, and nicotinic acid. The best source of this B-complex is sweet red table wines and especially dessert wines.

Although grapes are naturally rich in vitamin C, wine is not. Vitamin C oxidizes easily and most of it dissipates during the crushing and fermentation process.

For more than two thousand years, wine had been the universal solvent in pharmacy. It was not until Prohibition in the United States that standards for the various types of wine were eliminated from the pharmacopoeia. Although wine is not officially listed in the National Formulary or the U.S. Pharmacopoeia, some pharmaceutical companies have continued to use wine as the solvent for various tonics, vitamins, and stomach bitters.

There are many advantages of wine as a medium. Wine has a wide alcoholic concentration, ranging from 7 to 24 percent, and can therefore maintain many relatively insoluble substances in stable solution. Many of the therapeutic drugs that are commonly used today are highly soluble at the mildly acidic pH level of wine. The presence of the natural salts of sodium and potassium in wine acts as a buffering agent to help stabilize many of the pharmaceutical agents. Wine production today is a perfected science and therefore pharmaceutical manufacturers are able to order standard wines with specific composition. In addition, the natural aro-

CHEMICAL COMPONENTS OF TYPICAL TABLE AND DESSERT WINES

	Units	Dry Red Wine	Dry White Wine	Medium Sweet Sherry	Port	Rosé	Champagne
Calcium	mg/liter	62.0	63.0	60.0	57.0	70.0	67.0
Copper	mg/l	0.2	0.2	0.4	0.5	0.1	0.3
Iron	mg/l	6.0	4.7	2.5	3.5	3.0	7.5
Potassium	mg/l	794.0	780.0	757.0	939.0	673.0	740.0
Sodium	mg/l	85.0	113.0	78.0	94.0	160.0	68.0
Sulphur dioxide	mg/l	109.0	142.0	93.0	100.0	120.0	88.0
Ethanol	% (vol)	12.2	11.9	19.9	19.8	12.2	12.5
Higher alcohols	mg/l	298.0	254.0	401.0	384.0	249.0	246.0
Acetaldehyde	mg/l	46.0	91.0	55.0	68.0	80.0	83.0
pH	—	3.7	3.5	3.7	3.8	3.45	3.2
Acetic acid	mg/l	470.0	290.0	400.0	330.0	290.0	500.0
Tartaric acid	%	0.6	0.6	0.4	0.4	0.6	0.7
Hexases	%	0.2	0.3	3.1	11.7	1.12	1.5
Total esters	mg/l	280.0	244.0	419.0	305.0	260.0	191.0
Tannins	%	0.18	0.03	0.03	0.1	0.05	0.04

Source: Leake, C.D., and Silverman, M. Alcoholic Beverages in Clinical Medicine. Chicago: Year Book Medical Publishers, Inc., 1966.

matic constituents present in wine provide an inexpensive and healthy flavoring for medications.

The following table shows the major constituents of the most typical wines.

ALCOHOL CONTENT—A COMPARISON

Beer: Varies between 2 and 8%
2%   light Scandinavian and Russian *kvass*
3.2%   many light American and college campus beers
4.5%   most American beers
8%   especially strong beers

Cordials: Blackberry, Maraschino, Anisette, Curaçao vary between 25 and 40%.
Dessert or sweet wines: Sherry, port, or Muscatel are approximately 20%.
Dry wines: Natural and unfortified wines—for example, most American table wines—vary from 12 to 14%. Chianti, Burgundy, and Sauternes range from 8 to 12%.
Vermouth or other apéritif wines: 18%
Spirits: Whiskey, gin, vodka, rum, brandy, and liqueurs vary between 40 and 50%.

Special Note: It is important to understand that alcoholic content is measured in percentage by volume or the proportion of alcohol in the fluid volume. Natural fermentation automatically stops at 14 percent; therefore, fortified wines have either brandy or alcohol added. Beverages with a low alcohol percentage are produced by drawing off the liquid early in the fermentation process. In contrast, distillation allows for spirits with a high alcoholic content.

CHAPTER FOUR

HOW TO LIVE TO BE 100-PLUS

Vibrant good health, sexual virility, and long life go hand in hand. Man has sought the Fountain of Youth since the dawn of history. Ponce de Léon sought his fabled fountain in Florida; the Bolivian Indians made a secret elixir from thornless cactus, which was said to have life-extending powers; and in Switzerland a man named Spalenjer, a few years ago, claimed to have developed a serum that would prolong life up to 150 years.

Interest in new methods of preventing premature aging is as strong today as it was in the Stone Age. The earliest medical records reveal a variety of interesting herbs and potions used to retard aging and revitalize virility. A Hindu doctor in 1400 B.C. prescribed tiger's sex glands for impotence.

Today's men and women live in a youth-oriented society and are as preoccupied with premature aging and longer life as their ancestors. Medical science of the twentieth century is concentrating on preventing disease and prolonging man's life. Many interesting discoveries on longevity are being reported daily from around the world. Today in the Soviet Union, extensive research programs are focusing on longer life with special studies being carried out in the Caucasus where centenarians are not unusual. The Soviet physiologist Tarkhanov said: "The time will come when it will be a disgrace for a man to die less than one hundred years old."

In this section, we will examine how Europeans use wine to prevent premature aging and to live longer.

The Rhône Valley is steeped in history and was once a main center of worship for the Persian sun god Mithras. The majestic Rhône flows south from Lyon between the Massif Central and the foothills of the Alps. Several years ago, I followed the picturesque Route Nationale 7: the Rhône "corniche" on the right bank of the river, starting at Vienne and finishing my trip in Avignon.

In Vienne, with its great Roman theater and Gothic cathedral, I interviewed many Vignerons. I was curious because I had noticed in the area a large proportion of older men and women with surprising vitality. I was told that many of the older generation owe their vitality and youthful appearance to a local drink called "Pontius Pilate Water," after the one-time Roman governor of the city. I can't extol the virtues of this local secret brew enough, so try it yourself and see if the results are formidable.

PONTIUS PILATE WATER

1 teaspoon	fennel seeds
1 teaspoon	mace
1 teaspoon	mint, dried
1 teaspoon	cloves
1 teaspoon	anise seeds
1 teaspoon	ginger
1 teaspoon	caraway seeds
1 teaspoon	cinnamon
1 teaspoon	nutmeg
1 teaspoon	thyme, dried
1 gallon	Côtes du Rhône (12–14% alcohol)

1. Put herbs in a blender or food processor and pulverize.
2. Add powdered herbs to wine.
3. Let stand 14 hours, stirring occasionally.
4. Distill the liquid.
   - For a simple at-home still, pour the Pontius Pilate Water into your teakettle and slip a rubber tube over the spout. The other end of the tube should be inserted into a glass jar. Cover the tube with ice cubes. This will condense the steam from the kettle, and the liquid will then collect in the jar.

From Sweden come several interesting rejuvenation secrets. Swedes enjoy an international reputation for youth and beauty. They have been using large quantities of vitamin C for centuries. Rose hips, a staple food in Sweden, is the richest natural source of vitamin C. After extensive travels throughout the country, I found the Swedish "fountain of youth" is a simple rose hips and red wine tea.

Vitamin C has a stimulating effect on the adrenal glands, which secrete about thirty steroid hormones vital to keeping your body working at peak efficiency. Scientists agree that decreased hormone output is directly responsible for the symptoms of old age.

Try including a Swedish rose hips soup or tea in your daily diet. Swedish Youth Tea should be considered an essential rejuvenating tonic for anyone over forty.

SWEDISH ROSE HIPS SOUP

For each serving put 2 tablespoons of rose hip powder in a cup of water. Bring to a boil, remove from heat, and steep for 5 minutes. Add ½ cup dry red wine, 1 teaspoon honey, and ½ tablespoon corn starch to thicken. Return to heat and boil for 3–5 minutes. Serve warm or chilled, sprinkled with wheat germ or sunflower seeds.

YOUTH TEA

Use 2 tablespoons of either rose hips powder or dried rose hips for each cup of water. Bring the mixture just to a boil and remove from heat immediately—*do not let boil*. Add 2 tablespoons red wine and let steep for 5 minutes for powder, or 15 minutes for whole dried halves. Strain; sweeten with honey if desired.

When making Swedish Youth Tea, aluminum utensils should be avoided. Scandinavian rose hips are available in the United States, in both whole or powdered form at most health food stores.

Whey is another Swedish secret for staying young. Whey is the clear liquid which separates from the curd when milk is curdled. In Sweden, whey cheese and whey butter are staple foods. In the United States, whey can be found in health food stores in either powder or tablets. In whey therapy, you can look and feel ten years younger in a surprisingly short time. Whey should be included in your daily diet. Follow the recommended dosage on the particular brand available in your area.

WHEY FACIAL

Mix together 1 teaspoon each of whey, white wine, and honey. Rub the mixture on your face, let dry, then rinse with warm water for a rosy, radiant, young complexion. Vitamin E in Sweden is commonly known as the "sex vitamin" and is sold in automatic dispensers.

A Japanese doctor, M. Higuchi, has shown that there is a definite relationship between youth and the continued, normal, healthy functioning of the sex glands. A vitamin E deficiency can reduce the hormone production of the sex glands and premote premature aging. To maintain a normal hormone level and insure potency, add the Vitality Plus drink to your daily diet.

VITALITY PLUS

¼ cup	sunflower seeds
2 tablespoons	soya milk powder
4	dates
¼ teaspoon	honey
2 cups	water
¼ cup	red wine
Vitamin E capsules—100 units	

1. Grind the seeds in a blender.
2. Add the remaining ingredients and liquefy.
   - Drink one cup of mixture daily, adding 100 units of vitamin E.

Bulgarians live longer and have a greater number of centenarians than any other country. Extensive research has led scientists to believe that their sour milk-oriented diet is responsible for their longevity. In a study, the Swedish doctor

E. M. Hoppe, questioning 158 Bulgarians one hundred years old or older, found that yogurt, kefir, and fermented foods were the dietary secret responsible for the Bulgarians' long and healthy life!

The famous Russian bacteriologist, Ilja Metchnikoff, in his book *How to Prolong Life* stated that the putrefaction of waste products in the large intestine is the major cause of premature aging. Dr. Metchnikoff felt that by preventing the development of toxins and the resulting self-poisoning in the colon, the normal life span could be successfully doubled.

After studying the long-living Bulgarians, who consume more yogurt than any other national group, Metchnikoff recommended the daily addition of soured milk products, such as yogurt and kefir, to help prevent intestinal putrefaction. Yogurt and other soured milk products contain lactose, a natural food to help promote the growth of friendly intestinal bacteria.

HOMEMADE YOGURT

It is important to use freshly made natural yogurt in your daily diet. If you don't have a yogurt-maker, try this simple, inexpensive recipe:

Take one quart skim milk and heat until almost but not quite boiling. Add 3 tablespoons yogurt starter, which you can buy at a health food store. Stir well. Pour mixture into a wide-mouthed thermos bottle. Cover and let stand overnight. In about 6–8 hours, your yogurt will be ready.

SWEDISH YOGURT DRINK

2 cups	plain yogurt
2 cups	fresh milk
½ cup	sweet red wine
2 tablespoons	wheat germ
1 tablespoon	honey
1 tablespoon	molasses

1. Combine the above ingredients.
2. Chill before serving.

BULGARIAN YOGURT BREW

Try this traditional summer drink, a favorite in Bulgaria and other Near Eastern countries.

Dilute yogurt with an equal quantity of either white or red wine. Season with a pinch of salt. Drink an 8 oz. glass daily.

During the sixteenth century, the French Emperor Francis I had been ill for many months with an unexplained illness. The court doctors were puzzled. A visiting doctor from Constantinople asked if he could try a "secret medicine": that medicine was yogurt. In the times before antibiotics, the health-giving bacteria produced in yogurt were considered a "miracle drug." Since the time of Francis, the French have called yogurt "lait de la vie éternelle" (milk of eternal life).

For your own "secret miracle," eat one cup of plain yogurt daily. Add two tablespoons red wine to the yogurt and let it stand overnight. Mix well in the morning and eat for breakfast.

Moslems in the Caucasus mountains of eastern Europe kept the method of preparation of their wonder food, kefir, secret because they believed that if the world knew it, kefir might lose some of its special power. They called this miraculous food "the grain of the prophet," although the word "kefir" probably is derived from the Turkish word "klif" which means "a good feeling," which it seems to produce in everyone who eats it.

Marco Polo brought samples of kefir back to the Western World in the thirteenth century, but it wasn't until the early nineteenth century that European doctors began to use kefir in the treatment of tuberculosis. High in B-vitamins and beneficial bacteria, and containing some alcohol, kefir has been found to have surprising curative effects on the digestive and eliminative tracts.

HOMEMADE KEFIR

Add 1 tablespoon of kefir grains to a glass of milk. Stir and let stand overnight at room temperature. The kefir is ready when the milk coagulates. Kefir is about 1–1.5 percent alcohol. The longer it stands before using the more alcohol is produced.

- Kefir grains are available at health food stores or by mail from R. A. J. Biological Laboratory, 35 Park Avenue, Blue Point, NY 11715

BULGARIAN KEFIR: ELIXIR OF YOUTH

Marinate a peach half in red wine overnight. Slice and add to 1 cup of homemade kefir. The fresh fruit may be seasonally changed to add variety, but the wine is essential to the detoxification process.

KEFIR YOUTH MASK

Combine 1 tablespoon kefir yeast with spring water to make a paste. Carefully spread paste on face in rotating motions, avoiding sensitive eye area. Lie down with feet elevated for 20 minutes until mask dries. Rinse off with warm water.

In the Middle East, sesame seeds are a staple. They are a natural wonder food, rich in calcium, protein, magnesium, potassium, lecithin, B-vitamins, and are an excellent source of vitamin E. Women have eaten halvah to restore their youth and sex appeal for generations. Halvah is essentially made from sesame seeds and honey, but the recipe I have included uses a sweet red wine. The recipe was given to me several years ago by a model in Paris who swore by its powers. If her radiant beauty was any indication of success, I'm convinced.

HALVAH

1 cup	sesame seeds
2 teaspoons	sweet red wine
2 teaspoons	honey

1. Grind the seeds in a blender.
2. Pour the powder into a small bowl.
3. Add the wine and let stand for 10 minutes.

4. Knead the honey into the mixture until the consistency of a hard dough is reached.
5. Roll into small balls.
   - Eat 1 a day.

CHAPTER FIVE

WINE AND SEX

A Roman, encamped along the Rhine, wrote, "Wine has three grapes—the first brings sensual pleasures, the second brings intoxication, the third, the offense."

Is wine an aphrodisiac? The answer is a definite yes. Psychologists and marriage counselors agree that one or two glasses of wine help people unwind, step out of their "civilized" image, and begin to feel.

In interviews with one hundred wine drinkers, I asked how wine affected their sex lives.

WOMEN

- "Two glasses of wine definitely make me more amorous."
- "A glass of wine relaxes me so I feel more open, giving, loving."
- "Red wine, especially Burgundy, makes my skin flush, my blood boil. It makes me horny."
- "Champagne makes me feel feminine, a seductress. I'm definitely more creative in bed."
- "Since I've been drinking wine beforehand, I experience the most wildly beautiful climaxes."
- "Wine is a definite turn-on."

All agreed that a glass or two of wine before making love enhanced their performance, made them more amorous and—in many cases—adventurous, but hard liquor and drunkenness were a definite deterrent to sex, making it ugly and unappealing.

MEN

- "Wine releases my inhibitions without making me lose my head."
- "Wine has improved my sex life. I have a tendency to come too fast, but after two glasses of wine I slow down and give my wife some pleasure."
- "Wine is the best turn-on I've ever found."
- "Wine has turned me into a more sexual person; screwing stoned isn't a lasting experience."
- "My wife and I share a bottle of wine in bed together three times a week—our sex life has never been so good and we just celebrated our thirtieth wedding anniversary."
- "Sex is sensitive, the ultimate feeling experience. Wine lets me relax, enjoy it more."

I am by no means advocating heavy drinking as a cure-all for sexual problems, but wine, taken in moderation, shared with your partner, can improve the libido and transform the sex act into an incredible experience.

APHRODISIACS

Aphrodite, goddess of love and beauty, has promoted romance since ancient times. The early Greeks believed that special foods, herbs, and wines created virility and success in love.

Many men now take daily vitamin E capsules to increase their sexual prowess, believing great lovers are made, not born. Is this method more effective than many of the historically proven powerful sexual stimulants? Maybe not, but why decide before trying a wide variety of sensuous delights available to you that may turn you on sexually—more than you could have ever imagined?

ROMAN LOVE POTION

Famed for reinforcing sexuality, this potion has helped stimulate the reluctant lover for centuries. Combine 1 quart of dry sherry with 3 tablespoons sugar, the juice of 2 oranges, 1 teaspoon grated orange rind, ½ teaspoon cinnamon and 1 teaspoon nutmeg. Simmer for 1–2 minutes and serve warm.

THE FABLED FIG

The fabled nomadic lovers of the desert relied on the secret of the fig to preserve their potency. Figs are rich in silicon, a mineral which prevents impotence. In France, men eat figs soaked in Champagne as a titillating dessert. Try marinating 1 pound of figs for 2 hours in a bottle of Champagne. Serve in a large wine glass. Eat slowly with your fingers.

SWEDISH LOVE RUB

From Sweden comes a potent brew guaranteed to light a fire in your skin. The ancient formula is said to bring exciting amour to those who massage it into their skin. Rub it on yourself, then slowly, sensually, on your lover.

1 pint	rose water
1 pint	red wine
2 tablespoons	dried mint
1½ cups	dried rosemary leaves
2 tablespoons	fresh grated lemon peel
2 tablespoons	fresh grated orange peel

1. Combine the rose water and wine in a covered container.
2. Add the other ingredients and marinate for one month.
3. Strain out the herbs.
   * Slowly rub the liquid over your skin. It's heavenly, sensuous, and oh, so sexy.

HEAVENLY HONEY

Honey ranks high on the foods list of aphrodisiacs and for centuries has been considered a powerful sexual stimulant. For a thrill, try this sensuously delightful taste treat:

¾ cup	honey
¾ cup	almond meal
2 cups	dry red wine
2	egg yolks
¼ teaspoon	ground nutmeg
1 tablespoon	arrowroot

1. Warm the honey until it bubbles slowly.
2. Beat together the almond meal, wine, egg yolks, and nutmeg.
3. Slowly blend the two mixtures together.
4. Dissolve the arrowroot in a small amount of red wine until a paste is formed.
5. Blend well into the honey and wine mixture.
6. Heat slowly until it thickens and serve in warmed glasses.

ROMAN SURPRISE

Hot mint tea is as seductive to the Romans as Champagne is to the French, and millions of Romeos can't be wrong. To make your own pungent brew, crush fresh mint in the bottom of a glass and pour over it hot white wine to make a fragrant tea that is considered an important aphrodisiac around the Mediterranean.

ORANGE SURPRISE

Orange blossoms and love have been synonymous for centuries as a symbol of undying emotion. Although Americans have always associated the orange blossom with restrained passion, Europeans have stepped up the tempo and proven the seductive power of the blossom. For an exciting dessert or enticing breakfast treat try this:

3 cups	fresh orange juice
1 teaspoon	arrowroot
3 tablespoons	cold dry white wine
½ cup	orange blossom honey
2 teaspoon	fresh grated orange rind

1. Heat orange juice.

2. Combine arrowroot and wine, add to juice, and cook until clear.

3. Add orange peel to honey and stir into juice.

4. Chill and mix with an equal amount of very dry Champagne.

THE SEDUCTIVE APPLE

The apple has been the source of temptation since Eve seduced Adam in the Garden. Aside from its high vitamin content, the apple is rich in magnesium and sulphur which directly stimulate the glands, relaxing the body, leaving it receptive to sexual response. The French eat their apples soaked in dry white wine, the Germans in brandy, and the Italians marinate them in honey and red wine.

THE EXOTIC OYSTER

Although scheming or planning may seem far from romantic, there is no denying the powerful effect oysters have on stimulating hormone production. A seductive hostess, anticipating an amorous evening, might consider including oysters broiled with sea kelp on her menu. The Portuguese marinate their oysters in equal portions of brandy and white wine before cooking, which intensifies their iodine content, insuring a smashing evening.

THE LOVE BATH

Combine equal quantities of dried honeysuckle, jasmine, fuchsia, carnation, and orange peel, one to two teaspoons of each depending on desired scent. Marinate in 1 quart of warm red wine for several hours. Pour into a steaming bath. The scent is wonderful, aromatic. Take a friend.

THE LOVE SCENT

Knut Larsson, the noted Swedish doctor at the University of Gothenberg has proved that the genital nerves and the olfactory nerves are in some way related—in other words, there is a definite physiological connection between sexuality and odor. The French biologist Marguerite Maury has proved the power of aromatherapy. Several famous establishments around the world provide a full service aroma massage. If you're in the area, try the Aroma Salons in London and Paris, the Essential in Beverly Hills, and the Renaissance in the Bahamas. If you don't travel in the jet set, try creating your own aroma salon at home by converting your bathroom using a hot plate or electric skillet:

Run a hot bath. On a hot plate or in a skillet heat ½ cup coconut oil, 1 cup red wine, and 1 teaspoon each of ginseng and rosemary. Simmer and simply inhale the vapor for 10 minutes. Then add mixture to bath and soak. If you are bathing with a friend, after 15 minutes you will be ready to retire to the bedroom. (Or, if you like to live dangerously, why move at all?)

CHAPTER SIX

WINE THERAPY: PREVENTION, TREATMENTS, AND CURES WITH WINE

The ways in which wine has been used to treat various physical disorders are indeed myriad. Currently, doctors are exploring the therapeutic uses of wine with increasing confidence and enthusiasm. They are prescribing it in the treatment of a wide spectrum of complaints ranging from anxiety to weight control and heart disease. In this chapter the illnesses that can potentially be alleviated by wine therapy are discussed in alphabetical order.

It is important to remember that *wine, like any drug, must never be used as medication without the knowledge and approval of your physician.* See the table of alcohol and drug interactions in Appendix A for the possible consequences of mixing wine and medicines improperly. And, of course, wine used in excess can be damaging to the health. Keeping these cautions in mind, let us look at the amazingly varied and numerous beneficial uses of wine.

ANXIETY

Who hasn't experienced "the lump" in the throat that feels as if you will choke with the next swallow? Research has shown that as the anxieties of the day increase, the throat tightens and by dinner has reached a climax.

Heavier red wines, higher in alcoholic content, are very successful in relieving stress. Try two glasses of a Médoc or Bordeaux with meals, especially at lunch; they will help alleviate the increased tensions of the afternoon.

Since biblical times, wine had been used as a tranquilizer, sedative, and anesthetic. The Romans filled a small cloth bag with thyme and soaked it in a dry, light, white wine. The herbed wine, taken three to four times per day, proved an excellent cure for nervous anxiety and digestion. I must admit that I have not tried this specific folk remedy, but the thought does sound intriguing.

Today the medical community understands the levels on which wines tranquilize.

- As a *tranquilizer,* wine reduces anxiety, and nervous and muscular tension, by acting as a mild depressant.
- As a *sedative,* wine relaxes, blotting out the aggression and excitement of the day.
- As a *hypnotic-sedative,* wine reinforces the historic use in large doses as an effective anesthesia. Therefore, as with all alcoholic beverages, caution and moderation must be used.

Physicians have found that relatively large doses of wine—three to four glasses—before bed cause significant emotional tension release and are extremely effective in treating "executive syndrome" skin irritations. In today's success-oriented society stress-related skin diseases appear in many different forms. The most characteristic is the rash composed of tiny red spots that develop into itchy blisters. These sores can either be dry or oozing depending on the amount of stress.

Light white wines are highly recommended, because of their high sulphur and manganese content. The usual dosage varies, depending on personal tolerance, between one-quarter and one-half liter per day consumed with meals.

Many patients have also found relief by combining equal quantities of the wine and water mixture as a poultice. The irritated area should be soaked two or three times per day until the swelling is reduced.

For normal anxiety release, it is important to consider not only which wine, but when wine is consumed. If the wine is drunk on an empty stomach, four ounces may be adequate, but taken with a meal eight ounces may be necessary to achieve the same results. The rate of alcohol absorption into the blood is critical in wine therapy. On an empty stomach the process takes approximately sixty minutes, but with a full stomach the absorption is much slower. Alcohol reaches its highest point in the blood between two and five hours after ingestion but remains effective for from ten to twelve hours.

THE TRANQUILIZER HABIT— IS THERE ANOTHER ANSWER?

Last year, more than 68 million prescriptions were written for Valium and Librium, which comprise almost 90 percent of the tranquilizer market. Fifteen percent of all adult Americans take Valium regularly, despite well-known agonizing withdrawal symptoms. At a Senate hearing in 1979 on the use and misuse of tranquilizing drugs, a young doctor testified, that "Withdrawal felt like 'somebody poured kerosene under my skin and then put a torch to me.'" Granted, not everyone experiences such terrifying symptoms, but each tiny pill increases dependence, either emotional or physical, and withdrawal at some stage is inevitable.

Over half of all tranquilizers prescribed are for stress-related problems, usually relatively minor emotional or physical problems—insomnia, lower-back pain, marital problems, headaches, and financial or job-related stress. In the majority of cases, they only mask the symptoms, postponing the inevitable—solving or facing the problem.

Doctors are gradually becoming more aware of the dangers of continued tranquilizer therapy. Barbara Gordon, in her best-selling book *I'm Dancing as Fast as I Can*, described with frightening reality her "cold turkey" withdrawal from Valium. Gordon was originally given Valium for lower-back pain, and like so many others, never went off the drug.

I am not disputing the fact that mood-altering drugs are beneficial in the treatment of severe psychological disorders. However, the problem we are dealing with here is over-prescription/overuse leading to dependence in order to cope with the ordinary stresses of everyday life—fights, anxieties, money problems. America has turned into a pill-popping nation, but it's not too late to take an interest in your body. Ask the doctor what that pill might do to you now as well as later, or, the most important question, do you have an alternative?

For centuries, wine has been used as a naturally mild and safe sedative. Medical experiments prove that the pharmacologic effects of wine are directly related to the proportion of alcohols and aldehydes. Two Yale scientists, L. A. Greenberg and J. A. Carpenter, conducting experiments under strictly controlled laboratory conditions, found that wine can significantly reduce emotional tension levels in human beings. Not only was wine effective in reducing anxiety levels associated with routine, everyday tension, but it was equally effective against sudden intense emotional stress.

The study also revealed that wine, when compared to other forms of alcohol, produced longer-lasting, more gradual relief, perhaps due to the natural buffering components of the wine combined with the relatively slow absorption rate from the digestive tract. Greenberg and Carpenter have concluded that the tension-relieving action of wine may explain "the considerable and universal use of this beverage in moderation, and the persistence of this use throughout the history of man."

FALLEN ARCHES AND TIRED FEET

While interviewing vineyard owners in northern Italy, I was told about an interesting and effective cure for fallen arches, a complaint that many grape harvesters contract after standing for years on uneven gravelly soil.

HERBAL FOOT LINIMENT

1½ ozs.	talcum powder
1 pint	strong red wine
½ pint	rum

1. Combine talcum powder and wine.
2. Cover and let stand for 2 days.
3. Add rum, cover; let stand for 1 week.
4. Strain liquid and pour into a tightly capped bottle.
   - Rub the feet with the liniment 4 times a day and either bind with clean gauze or wear thick white cotton socks. Relief should be noticed within 1 to 2 weeks. Many

vineyard workers use this liniment as a prophylactic and to soothe tired feet.

BURNS

How bad is a burn? A first-degree burn is superficial and causes the skin to turn red. Second-degree burns are much deeper and cause the skin to split and blister. Third-degree burns destroy skin layers affecting the deeper tissues.

First- and second-degree burns are extremely painful but can usually be treated successfully at home. To minimize the amount of skin damage it is very important to apply something cold immediately.

BURN RELIEF

Prepare a mixture of equal quantities of red wine and cider vinegar and keep it in the refrigerator. Apply directly to the burn for 5 minutes until the pain is relieved. Continue the application for 1 hour if necessary or if the pain returns.

CORNS AND CALLUSES

Corns are usually caused by tight-fitting shoes and although not dangerous are extremely painful. If both corns and calluses are treated promptly they can be cured in a very short time.

Special note: Diabetics must never treat their own feet or take any medication before consulting a physician.

CORN REMOVAL

Soak the corn in warm water for 20 minutes. Immerse a corn pad in red wine then soak in a 10 percent solution of salicylic acid. Apply the corn pad for 4 days. Soak the foot again in warm water and the corn will come out easily.

CALLUS REMOVAL

Calluses can be removed by applying the above treatment and when soft gently pared down.

ARTHRITIS

WHAT IS ARTHRITIS?

There are over one hundred types of arthritis, but rheumatoid and osteoarthritis are responsible for over 90 percent of all cases. "Arth" means joint and "itis" means inflamed, thus true arthritic joints are red, warm, swollen, and painful to move.

Osteoarthritis is thought to be the result of "wear and tear" and is common in late middle-age due to a degenerative process in the joints. Rheumatoid arthritis affects all ages and is an extremely painful, crippling disease. Women contract rheumatoid arthritis at a rate three times higher than men.

WHAT CAUSES ARTHRITIS?

Arthritis is not a localized joint disease but a systemic disease that affects the entire body. Swollen, inflamed, painful joints are not the first sign of the onset of arthritis. For years the arthritic patient has been suffering from systemic disturbances stemming from digestive, glandular, and nutritional deficiencies. The underlying causes for the development of conditions leading to arthritis are still the subject of intense medical controversy.

European doctors feel the only way to obtain a lasting arthritis cure is to totally withdraw from all drugs and chemicals and adopt a biological treatment which allows the body's own healing forces to normalize the metabolic processes.

Therapeutic fasting in Europe is an important curative procedure in the treatment of arthritis. The famous grape cure fast for arthritis patients helps purify, cleanse, detoxify, and restore health.

THE EUROPEAN GRAPE CURE

Grapes, rich in enzymes and natural vitamins, are considered throughout Europe as a "life force," and a powerful catalyst in natural healing. Major health clinics in Europe offer especially designed one-, two-, or several-week grape cures. European physicians have recommended the unusual grape cure to arthritic patients with amazing success. The modified fasting procedure of the grape diet produces unusual curative properties that many physicians feel are directly linked to the noble fruit.

AT-HOME GRAPE CURE

Since most people are not able to travel to the various European clinics that offer the grape cure, I have outlined a simple at-home fasting program that can safely reproduce the famous European cure.

In Sweden, fasting is a national hobby. Thousands of Swedes fast every year for one or two weeks, as an effective method of cleansing the body, building resistances and stamina, and preventing illness.

Liquid, fruit, or juice fasting is not dangerous and the program can be safely followed at home, although you should *always consult a physician before undertaking any radical fasting or dieting.*

Contrary to common belief, fasting is not weakening or depleting. In fact, it produces total regeneration and rejuvenation of the body's functions.

To prepare yourself for the fast, a cleansing diet should be followed for two days. Eat only raw fruits and vegetables, alternating at each meal.

The day preceding the fast, do not eat dinner and take a dose of castor oil in the late afternoon, and an enema before going to bed. The enema solution should be a mild mixture of camomile tea added to a quart of warm water. Enemas are an important part of the fasting program. They help eliminate toxic waste material from the colon. Even after two weeks of fasting the amount of waste products that are eliminated is amazing.

After the system is prepared, eat nothing but grapes for two weeks. On the first day, begin slowly by eating only a few grapes for breakfast, increasing the number for lunch and eventually consuming two ounces for dinner. On the second day, eat three ounces for each meal. The third day, slowly increase the number of ounces, and from the fourth day you can eat as many grapes as you want, as long as you don't consume more than four pounds a day.

Drink only mineral water and only when you are thirsty.

HELPFUL HINTS

—Eat the grapes slowly, chew thoroughly.

—Eat grapes whole, including seeds and skins.

—Eat only very ripe grapes.

—Chew seeds, but do not swallow every one. Seedless grapes are allowed.

—Try buying grapes directly from orchards that have not been chemically fertilized. Supermarket grapes must be soaked and washed carefully to remove insecticides.

When the grape cure is completed follow the directions carefully for breaking a fast.

HOW TO BREAK A FAST

Breaking the fast is an extremely important part of the program. If it is done incorrectly, the beneficial effects of the fast can be totally destroyed.

The three main rules of breaking a fast are:

1. Chew the food slowly.
2. Don't overeat!
3. Make a slow transition back to your normal diet.

Day one: Eat one apple, a bowl of fresh vegetable soup, and as much fresh fruit juice as wanted.

Day two: Add to the above menu mashed potatoes and yogurt.

Day three: Eat raw vegetable salad, cooked rice, and fresh cottage cheese.

Day four: Start eating normally.

It is possible to find relief from the excruciating pain and discomfort of aching joints, arthritis, neuritis, and rheumatism by the use of special massage oils and lotions.

HUNGARY WATER

Legend says that in the thirteenth century Queen Elizabeth of Hungary became a prisoner to the paralysis of her joints. The court physicians prepared the following lotion, which she rubbed on several times daily until she was cured:

Combine 1 ounce of lavender, 1 ounce of rosemary, ½ ounce of myrtle with 1 quart of brandy and ¼ cup of red wine. Let the mixture steep for 2 weeks, then strain.

RHEUMATISM (ARTHRITIS)

Many arthritic patients call their red, stiffened, swollen joints rheumatism. The pain and suffering are the same, whatever it is called. Most physicians feel helpless when faced with an arthritic patient because there is no approved cure. But many people are now reappraising folk cures. Try this old English formula for the relief of arthritic pain:

ENGLISH ARTHRITIS REMEDY

Fill a quart bottle half-full with equal parts of the following herbs: wild cherry bark, prickly ash bark, and rattle root.

To the mixture add double the amount of sarsaparilla root and poplar. Add equal amounts of whiskey and red wine until the bottle is full. Let stand 1 week. Take 1 teaspoon before each meal.

ATHLETE'S FOOT

The dread foot fungus causes the skin between the toes to become unbearably itchy, cracked, and moist. Athlete's foot can be controlled by keeping the feet dry and changing their acid balance.

From France comes this remedy to warm the heart and soothe the feet of every itchy athlete.

WHITE WINE FOOT BALM

1 oz.	sage
1 oz.	agrimony
2 cups	white wine

1. Combine all the ingredients.
2. Heat for 20 minutes but do not let boil.
3. Keep covered.
   - When the mixture is cool enough for you to tolerate, soak your feet for as long as you can. Repeat several times a day.

THE FRENCH FIG ANTI-CANCER FACTOR

Since biblical times physicians have used the fig tree to cure a variety of disorders ranging from coughs to heart disease. Thomas Culpeper, the governor of Virginia in 1673, prescribed the milk of the leaves for wart removal. Today, many people still use the juice of a freshly marinated fig to remove warts and to ease painful skin ulcers and chronic sores.

In Austria figs are boiled with equal amounts of barley water and wine to produce a beverage effective in curing bronchial complaints.

Recent medical reports show that cancer is very rarely found in areas where figs are eaten daily. Based on his research, a French doctor, L. F. Bordas, believes that figs contain an anti-cancer factor which may help prevent cancerous conditions from developing.

CHAMPAGNE FIG MARINADE

Fill a large glass jar with fresh figs. Cover with Champagne or white wine and let stand for 2 weeks. Eat 2 or 3 of the figs daily.

COLDS, FLU, AND UPPER RESPIRATORY DISORDERS

So you have a runny nose, aches and pains, the shakes, and a scratchy voice. You watch in silence as everyone around you succumbs to the same symptoms. The doctor, with a general lack of enthusiasm, diagnoses the common cold or local bug. He may prescribe an antihistamine that will make you feel groggier than any "over-the-counter" cold medication, but nothing will shorten the illness. Many cold preparations cause alarming complications, and evidence indicates they not only do not help relieve symptoms, but may even prolong the illness. Most doctors recommend aspirin, lots of fluids, and rest.

The body requires extra fluid, especially if a fever is present. Fluids help keep the mucus liquid and prevent complications such as ear infection and bronchitis. A fever should never be ignored and should be treated promptly by your physician.

Champagne was added to the fevered patient's diet successfully for centuries before the discovery of aspirin. Dry or brut Champagne helps stimulate the body's natural defenses against fever. Both sulphur, in the form of potassium sulphate, which acts as a detoxifying agent in the body, and phosphorus are found in Champagne and are essential to the well-being of the feverish patient. If your doctor agrees, try combining Champagne therapy with the normally prescribed medication.

Personally, I am extremely sensitive to all medications and try to avoid pills whenever possible. Last winter, my daughter Michelle brought home from school the worst cold our family ever had, and it systematically made the rounds of everyone. Our doctor, knowing my sensitivity to medications, recommended Champagne therapy, and I am a confirmed convert. He prescribed one bottle of dry or brut Champagne per day, taken in small doses of one glass per hour. The cure was surprisingly successful. My fever broke within twelve hours, and I continued the treatment for two days, which helped considerably to relieve my aches and pains. My husband, who is the worst patient in the world, stayed with the traditional aspirin therapy and was still suffering days after I had recovered.

The French have an extraordinary natural cure for the flu. Several years ago, while visiting friends in the south of France, I came down with a seasonal case of influenza. I had never felt so weak or debilitated. My friends sent for the local doctor, a funny little man who had been treating the townspeople for more than forty years.

I lay there dreading the expected prescription of a massive dose of antibiotics. To my surprise, instead of a hypodermic needle, he pulled a bottle of Côtes du Rhône from his little black bag. He explained that the wine was not only high in alcoholic content but contained its own natural antibiotics that the system can tolerate without harmful side effects. He prescribed heating the contents of the bottle of wine in a double boiler to 140° F, adding five teaspoons of sugar, one slice of lemon peel, and one tablespoon of cinnamon, then simmering for three minutes. (Drink one full glass of the wine mixture four times a day; the therapy can be continued for three days.) I felt considerably better within two days, without any of the sick aftereffects of a bout of flu.

COLD REMEDIES

In Switzerland many physicians recommend a simple onion wine to relieve the symptoms of a cold. The procedure is simple: Cut a fresh raw onion in half; immerse in a large glass of hot water. Let stand for two to three seconds and then remove. Add two tablespoons of white wine. Sip the water throughout the day. I can personally attest that this cure has amazing results.

CHEST COLD REMEDY

For fast relief of bronchial congestion, try the following formula:

½ lb.	comfrey root
½ lb.	spikenard root
½ lb.	elecampane root
1 gal.	water
8 oz.	red wine
3 cups	honey

1. Add roots to water.
2. Boil until mixture is reduced to 1 quart.
3. Pour into ½-gallon bottle.
4. Add wine and honey.
   - Take 1 teaspoon every 2 hours.

HOARHOUND-WINE TEA

A hoarhound-wine tea has been used for centuries in France to help relieve coughs and bronchial congestion:

Brew a strong cup of hoarhound tea; sweeten it with 1 teaspoon of honey and add 1 tablespoon of Burgundy wine. Take a hot footbath, drink the tea, and go to bed. Cover yourself with several warm blankets. Within twelve hours you should notice free expectorant.

CATNIP TEA

Not only cats fall in love with catnip; you will, too, after seeing its beneficial effects in treating colds and hoarseness. Catnip is a very common plant that can be purchased at most health food stores.

Follow the directions on the package for making a hot tea. Drink it slowly while taking a very hot footbath. Follow by drinking 1 glass of warm water to which has been added 3 tablespoons of Rhine wine. The effects will be dramatic.

RED CLOVER-WINE TEA

For relief of upper respiratory infection, especially hoarseness, colds and coughs, try drinking red clover and wine tea.

Make 1 pint of strong tea and add ¼ cup of red wine. Keep this warm, and drink 1 mouthful every 1 to 2 hours.

ACUTE LARYNGITIS/SMOKERS' THROAT

Laryngitis or hoarseness is an irritation of the vocal cords. Many people suffer the most during the winter cold and flu season, but laryngitis can strike at any time so it's best to be prepared. Temporary, mild hoarseness is usually caused by a viral infection. Persistent or frequent hoarseness can have many causes and should be checked by your physician.

To treat the distressing hoarseness that may linger after an upper respiratory tract infection, try an old Italian cure that has saved many an opera star's career:

Mix 1 teaspoon of dry white wine, 1 teaspoon of vinegar, and 2 drops of honey in an 8-ounce glass of warm water. Drink the mixture every hour for several hours. By the last dose there should be a noticeable improvement. This is also a very effective precautionary measure for irritated smokers' throat.

SORE THROAT

For relief of chronic sore throats try the following mixture:

Fill a pint bottle half-full with powdered prickly ash. Add equal amounts of whiskey and Burgundy wine until full. Cover and let stand for 7 days. Take 1 teaspoon 4 times a day. The mixture may be made in advance and kept until needed.

SINUS INFECTIONS

If you have ever suffered from a severe sinus infection, you know true misery. Your nose becomes clogged, you can't breathe or smell, and your face swells and your head aches. Your one thought is relief.

Most physicians prescribe long and sometimes dangerous courses of antibiotics. While visiting a friend several years ago in Vienna, my sinuses began to act up. She took me to her family physician, a Russian, who prescribed an extraordinary herbal cure:

GARLIC SURPRISE

Through a garlic press mash two large garlic cloves into a glass. Add 20 drops of water and 20 drops of white wine. Let the mixture stand for 20 minutes. Shake well. Strain and use only clear liquid. Incline your head and put 10 drops of liquid in each nostril. Close each nostil with fingertips and sniff.

- Don't be surprised at the initial intense burning; it should only last several seconds, then the dam will burst with bright red flares. The results are amusing, and the inflammation should have been greatly reduced within 3 days. I was most surprised that I did not reek of garlic, but the doctor explained that it was absorbed by the infection.

HERPES SIMPLEX

Herpes simplex, also known as cold sores or fever blisters, is caused by a virus. A herpes attack can be triggered by a variety of causes ranging from too much sun to poor nutrition.

While in Switzerland, I met a doctor in Gstaad who treated herpes sufferers by soaking fresh yellow apple slices in white wine for an hour, then applying the slices to the inflamed area.

I must admit that I have never tried this method for a cold sore, but I have found it very effective against severely chapped "skier's lips."

WINE AND THE DIABETIC

Diabetes is a disorder of the metabolism in which the body is unable to convert carbohydrates into usable energy, creating an excess of sugar in the blood and urine.

Diabetes is not a new disease; even the early Greeks were familiar with the distinctive symptoms of excessive thirst, uncontrollable hunger, and increased urination. Combined, these symptoms cause a debilitation of the body often complicated by mental depression.

Today, diabetes can be successfully treated by three different techniques, depending on the severity of the case. Many times mild cases only require strict dietary control, while more complicated cases utilize an oral therapeutic medication, and severely advanced cases require insulin injections.

But before 1922 and the discovery of insulin, physicians, especially in Europe, relied heavily on wine for diabetic treatment. Although it is inadvisable now to rely solely on alcohol as a medication, the diabetic can benefit by the addition of wine to his dietary program.

Many physicians are regularly incorporating dry table wines in the diabetic diet. These wines play an important role in maintaining both the physiological and psychological well-being of the patient. Unfortunately, a small percentage of doctors in the United States still believe in the Prohibition spirit and refuse to prescribe wine to their diabetic patients despite positive clinical research. Tests prove that a diabetic can drink as much as twenty-four ounces of dry wine without any significant blood sugar elevation.

Most diabetic diets are bland and uninteresting. It is difficult to plan a gourmet meal solely around the diabetic's inability to tolerate sugar. Wine provides the patient with a good-tasting, interesting source of calories that are not dependent on insulin for use.

Wine is ideal for the diabetic not just because it enhances a rather Spartan diet, but due to the slow rate of its absorption from the digestive tract, which produces low blood-alcohol concentrations, and allows for a more predictable calorie count. In addition, studies prove that when wine and no other form of alcoholic beverage is taken with a meal the blood sugar level is lower in the veins than in the capillary blood vessels.

Wine produces energy that is not converted by the body into fat. More importantly, wine alcohol is not converted into unneeded fatty acids or glucose.

Scientists are still studying the total effect of wine on the diabetic, but it is already known that wine in moderate amounts decreases the blood sugar level in diabetics, while having no apparent effect on nondiabetics. Researchers are now trying to isolate a substance suspected to be in grapes that has the same effect as insulin on carbohydrate metabolism.

The amount of wine to be included in the diabetic diet must be calculated by a physician, as both the caloric and sugar content of the specific wine must be incorporated in the diet plan. A medical study of the effects of calorically equivalent amounts of ethanol and dry wine on plasma lipids, ketones and blood sugar in diabetic and nondiabetic subjects found that in certain patients wine calories can be substituted for fat calories in the exchange system used in calculating the diabetic diet. Only the attending physician, who is familiar with the patient's life-style and individual metabolic characteristics, is qualified to make these calculations.

The correct choice of wine is essential to the success of the program. Unfortunately, American wines generally do not list sugar content on the label as many European wines do, but the residual sugar content of most dry table wines is normally only 1.5 percent or less. Fortunately for the diabetic, many wines are included in this category.

RECOMMENDED WHITES	RECOMMENDED REDS
CHABLIS	CABERNET SAUVIGNON
CHARDONNAY	CHIANTI
GREEN HUNGARIAN	CLARET
RIESLING	GAMAY
SAUVIGNON	PINOT NOIR
SYLVANER	ZINFANDEL
TRAMINER	

Leake and Silverman, in their book *Alcoholic Beverages in Clinical Medicine*, defined the sugar content (in grams) of wines in an average four-ounce serving as: 0.3 in dry red table wines, 0.4 in dry white table wines, 1.3 in rosé table wines, 1.8 in Champagne, and 4.9 or sometimes more in sweet white table wines and Kosher wines. In two ounces of apéritif or dessert wine the values were: 1.2 grams for dry sherry, 1.9 grams for medium sherry, and 6 grams or more for port, Muscatel and sweet sherry.

An interesting medical study was conducted on Italian and Italian-American adults that suggests a relationship between the regular daily consumption of wine and the prevention of diabetes.

In the study, 480 subjects were randomly selected, of whom 73 were diabetic—15 overt and 58 with borderline diabetic glucose tolerance curves. These subjects proved to be total abstainers or extremely light drinkers, while the remaining 407 subjects consumed large quantities of wine daily and had normal glucose tolerance curves.

THE DIGESTIVE SYSTEM

Digestion is one of the most important processes of the body. Poor digestion is an integral part of our busy everyday life. It was once thought that male executives had an edge on the market, but in today's changing work force, blue-collar workers and women are popping more and more antacid tablets.

The two-martini lunch is a disaster for the stomach. Bottled mineral water, which has taken the country by storm, provides little more help as most carbonated waters are artificially produced and provide very few natural chemical elements that aid digestion. Wine, on the other hand, is the only natural beverage that closely resembles gastric juice. When taken in reasonable amounts, it increases salivation, gently stimulates gastric acidity aiding in digestion, and natural evacuation. Four ounces of an apéritif wine—for example, dry sherry taken twenty minutes before a meal—is sufficient to stimulate gastroenteric actions and appetite, while eight ounces of a dry table wine is adequate if consumed with a meal. Alcohol in high concentrations may irritate the delicate gastric mucus, but wine has been proved to be beneficial to gastric activity.

Chronic poor digestion is directly linked to insufficient digestive juices, poor gastric muscle tone, or a combination of both. Dry Champagne has a favorable pH and so one or two glasses of it after meals has been prescribed for centuries to relieve digestive troubles. The tannins, glucides, and natural carbon dioxide help strengthen muscle tone, and aid in the absorption of hard-to-digest albuminoid substances such as meat and fish.

Wine is especially helpful in the care of patients whose digestive problems are influenced by emotional factors. It is important to note that while wine is beneficial to a wide variety of gastric problems, it is contraindicated in cases of gastric cancer, pyloric stenosis, gastritis, and suspected gastric hemorrhage.

In the case of either a duodenal or chronic gastric ulcer there is no standard practice, and it is best to consult your doctor on an individual basis. If the ulceration is acute, wine is contraindicated, but after healing has begun, wine can produce a mild tranquilization that is usually beneficial without causing any local irritation. Due to the favorable pH, one glass of dry Champagne, taken during a meal, is usually prescribed.

The hiatus hernia, a protrusion of a small part of the stomach through an opening at the base of the esophagus, is a product of our affluent, lazy society. It affects 40 percent more women than men, and is usually corrected by a regimen of exercise and diet, depending on the amount of digestive impairment. A medium dry Champagne, with its high potassium content, which helps restore muscle tone and flexibility, is desirable. One to two glasses taken with small meals have proved successful in treatment.

The malabsorption syndrome, a functional disorder of the small intestine that often follows gastric and intestinal surgery, can be effectively treated with dry white wines. In malabsorption, the small intestine is impaired or completely unable to absorb the normal amount of nutrients and fats from foods. The malabsorption syndrome is found in regional enteritis, tuberculosis, malignancies, and when half or more of the small intestine has been removed or received massive exposure to X-ray. The malabsorption syndrome is often seen in aging men and women when mineral oil has been used constantly as a laxative. When white wine is used to relieve discomforts after surgery, fat absorption is restored to normal without increased gastric distress. One to two glasses of a dry white table wine with meals is recommended.

The tannin content of wine provides an excellent treatment for irritable colon, which is attacking with more frequency our anxiety-ridden population. The symptoms are varied and can imitate every digestive disease known, but are usually accompanied by spasmodic abdominal pains. One to two glasses of a dry white wine that is low in alcohol content balance the tone of the intestine and mildly tranquilize the emotions, which help control intestinal spasms.

Constipation, on the other hand, is due to sluggishness, not hyperactivity, and can be induced by dependence on laxatives and enemas from childhood. The colon is very sensitive and responds to nervous factors, fear, anxiety, and continuous haste.

Wine can be successfully used to help the sluggish digestive system. One to two glasses at mealtime of a slightly sweet white wine that is low in alcohol but rich in tartrates, the principal acid of wine, and glycerine will help to gently stimulate the intestine. The French Rosé d'Anjou or Vouvray are excellent, as is the California Grenache Rosé.

Diarrhea, better known by travelers to Mexico as "Montezuma's Revenge," is usually caused by a mild bacterial infection. Some people are more sensitive than others, and attacks can be either acute and momentary, or chronic. Travelers in less developed countries should avoid drinking the water entirely. The known antibacterial properties of wine make drinking one to two glasses of your favorite wine daily advisable as a protective measure. If an acute attack develops, two glasses of a light red Beaujolais accompanied by a bland diet are usually helpful.

Chronic diarrhea should be treated by your doctor, but many physicians agree that red wine, especially the Médocs or Napa Cabernet, are beneficial in relieving diarrhea because

60

of the amount of tannin contained in the wine. Try one glass before and after each meal for relief.

Patients suffering from enteritis, a painful inflammation of the intestinal membranes accompanied by diarrhea, have recently been helped by including wine in their medical treatment and diet. Many doctors have found red wine, especially a Médoc or a Burgundy, useful in the treatment of enteritis.

CONSTIPATION REMEDY

Senna has been used in Oriental and European countries for safe, harmless relief of constipation for more than a thousand years:

For the correct dose, take 1 teaspoon of powdered senna followed by half a glass of warm water, to which has been added 1 tablespoon of Rhine wine, every 3 hours until relief is achieved.

BUTTERNUT LAXATIVE

Butternut is one of the most effective laxatives known:

Fill a quart bottle with small pieces of butternut. Add equal parts of whiskey and strong Burgundy wine. Cover and let stand for 2 weeks. Take 3 tablespoons a day until the bowels become regulated and loose. The mixture may be made in advance and stored until needed.

BITTERS FOR DIGESTION

Europeans strongly believe in bitters as a mild stomach tonic that promotes digestion and relieves indigestion.

Throughout the centuries local bitters formulas were closely guarded secrets handed down from generation to generation. Some well-known bitters brands include Fernet Branca and Unicum from Italy. Campari is another famous Italian bitters sold on an international scale as is Unterberg from Germany.

The following bitters recipes are little known but highly effective:

SWEDISH BITTERS

½ oz.	ground anise seed
½ oz.	ground coriander seed
½ oz.	ground gentian root
½ oz.	ground orange peel
½ oz.	ground cinchonic bark
½ oz.	ground cardamom seed
¼ oz.	ground gum kino
1 pt.	whiskey
1 qt.	dry red wine
3 qts.	water
1 lb.	sugar

1. Soak all the herbs in the alcohol for 1 week.
2. Pour off the liquid and reserve.
3. Add the dregs to 1 quart of water, boil for 1 minute, strain out the herbs.
4. Add the alcohol mixture, and the remaining water and sugar.
   • Take one wineglassful before each meal and at bedtime.

AUSTRIAN ALPINE BITTERS

1 oz.	centaury
2 ozs.	coriander seed
2 ozs.	chamomile
2 ozs.	sweet flag
3 ozs.	orange peel
4 ozs.	orris root
2 qts.	whiskey
1 pt.	dry red wine
3 pts.	water
4 ozs.	sugar

1. In a food processor combine all the herbs and grind until powdered.
2. In a large stainless-steel or enamel pan combine herbs, alcohol, water and boil for 10 minutes.
3. Add the sugar.
4. Store in tightly capped bottle.
   • Take 1 tablespoon 4 times a day.

GERMAN HOPS BITTERS

½ oz.	ground clove
1 oz.	cinnamon
2 ozs.	orange peel
2 ozs.	cardamom
4 ozs.	hops
1 cup	whiskey
1 qt.	dry sherry
1 cup	sugar
red wine	

1. In a blender, grind the herbs.
2. Marinate in the combined alcohol for 1 week.
3. In a large stainless-steel or enamel pan, boil for 5 minutes.
4. Add the sugar and enough red wine to make 1 gallon.
5. Store in a covered glass jar.
   • Take one wineglassful 3 times a day

INDIGESTION

For centuries the French have relied on a hot tansy and wine tea to relieve acid indigestion or severe stomach cramps, and to promote digestion.

Make a tansy tea by steeping dried tansy leaves in equal parts of water and red wine.

For chronic digestive problems a tansy tincture may be more effective. Fill a pint bottle one half full with powdered tansy. Add a mixture of equal amounts of red wine and whiskey. Cover and let stand for 7 days. Take 1 tablespoonful 3 times a day.

BLACK PEPPER TEA

To make 1 pint combine

1 teaspoon of black pepper and 1 teaspoon of red wine in a saucepan. Let stand for 5 minutes. Add 1 pint of boiling water. Swallow 1 mouthful of tea every 5 minutes until stomach pains are relieved.

OLD ALPINE CURE

To relieve that full, pressing, heavy weight sensation in the pit of the stomach, try this old Alpine cure:

In a pint bottle cut up a yellow dock root. Fill bottle with equal amounts of red wine and whiskey. Cover and let stand for 14 days. Take 1 tablespoon 2 to 3 times a day, preferably before meals.

HICCOUGHS

There must be thousands of different home remedies for curing hiccoughs, ranging from the ridiculous to the absurd. While at an elegant embassy dinner party in Bonn I was blessed with an embarrassing hiccough attack. My dinner partner, noticing my distress, excused himself and returned in a few minutes with a wineglassful of a colorless liquid. He told me to drink. Knowing he was an eminent doctor, I obeyed. Seconds later my hiccoughs had stopped, without my having to stand on my head while shaking my left foot or holding a brown paper bag over my face while counting backward from one hundred.

The secret is simple: In a glass combine two teaspoons of white or red wine with two teaspoons of cider vinegar.

FATIGUE

Swiss mountain climbers use a gentian wine mixture to relieve fatigue with exceptionally fast results. Many Europeans have found that the mixture is indispensable after a long trip when you arrive dead tired and feeling ill.

GENTIAN WINE TONIC

2 ozs.	crushed gentian root
1½ pts.	strong red wine

1. Combine ingredients in a covered glass container.
2. Let stand for 2–3 weeks.
   • Take 1 tablespoon when needed.

GLAUCOMA

Glaucoma is one of the most important causes of blindness in middle age, affecting more than 1.5 million people in the United States.

The disease causes vision impairment due to a rise in the fluid pressure within the eye. Wine therapy has been successfully used to reduce the pressure of the intraocular fluid. This process is accomplished by suppressing the normal hormone that eliminates unnecessary fluid from the body.

Acute glaucoma today is being treated with increased success by surgical procedures, but chronic glaucoma still may only be treated with medication. Many physicians find that the addition of wine to the chronic glaucoma patient's diet is very beneficial.

Every glaucoma patient should be aware of how alcohol—and especially wine—can help avert tragedy.

Glaucoma victims who find themselves without medication can safely substitute wine or other alcoholic beverages and avoid serious consequences. Clinical tests show that one pint of wine will, within one hour, reduce intraocular pressure to a safe level. The pressure will remain normal for from four to five hours. If wine, which is considered the best emergency medication, is not available, one liter of beer or one-half cup of whiskey may be substituted.

Wine is also being used successfully for pre-surgery glaucoma patients who are sensitive to the essential pressure-reducing drugs. The point should be stressed, though, that wine should never be taken four to five hours before an eye examination, because the intraocular pressure will be abnormally low, providing a false test reading.

HEART AND RELATED DISORDERS

THE CURRENT SCOREBOARD

During the past fifty years, coronary disease has increased in the United States by five hundred percent. Today, an estimated 30 million Americans suffer from some form of heart or blood vessel disease. This year, an estimated one million people will have heart attacks; 650,000 of those will die, and 200,000 will be between the ages of forty-five and sixty-five.

The statistics sound grim, but Americans have an outstanding aptitude for survival, and a healthy upswing is under way. Medical experts are just now beginning to see the full impact of our changing life-styles.

The American heart disease rate is still one of the highest in the world, but doctors believe that preventive measures combined with a healthier life-style can eventually overcome cardiovascular disease.

Wine and brandy have played an important role in treating and preventing cardiovascular disease since the thirteenth century. The alcohols and aldehydes in wine have been clinically proven to have a direct relaxing effect on the cardiovascular system.

Because of its relatively low alcohol content, wine makes a more advisable relaxant than stronger spirits. Many people have the mistaken impression that the alcohol content of wine alone is responsible for producing the advantageous effects, but in fact it is the combination of the alcohol and the complex chemical composition of the nonalcoholic components.

Daily wine consumption can help in the prevention and treatment of arteriosclerosis. The French doctor J. Masquelier has reported that the complex phenolic substances found in wines, such as leucoyanidin, isoquercitroside, and epicatichin, have proved to aid in reducing blood-cholesterol levels.

Recent medical evidence strongly suggests that moderate daily consumption of wine may prevent coronary disease, even when the diet is high in fats and cholesterol.

Wine has been used in effectively controlling the severity of angina pectoris attacks or even preventing the attacks entirely. As a natural pain reliever, wine has been used successfully in treating diseases such as Buerger's disease, Raynaud's disease, and arteriosclerosis with thrombosis.

Wine can be successfully prescribed to reduce the apprehension and general discomfort associated with high blood pressure.

Next to accidental death, heart disease is still the number-one killer in the United States, and accounts for one out of three deaths each year.

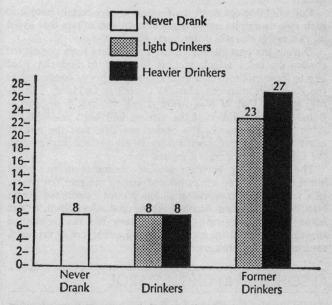

CORONARY HEART DISEASE RATES IN MEN AGED 45–59 AT THE START OF THE TECUMSETT STUDY BY DRINKING PATTERN

Never Drank

Light Drinkers

Heavier Drinkers

Coronary heart disease defined as myocardial infarction. Lighter drinking defined for this analysis as 4 ounces of absolute alcohol per week (about 10 ounces of distilled spirits) or less, heavier drinking as any larger amount.*

This study is most interesting in that there was no significant difference in the heart attack rate in drinkers and non-drinkers aged forty-five to fifty-nine, but former drinkers were three times more likely to have a heart attack. Question: Why do former drinkers run a greater risk of heart attack? Could the cessation of drinking accelerate blood cholesterol levels?

*From *Alcohol and Health*, U.S. Department of Health, Education, and Welfare, 1959.

Although we are learning more about preventing heart disease, the age-old question of why certain people develop heart disease and have heart attacks is still something of a mystery. Scientists have been successful in isolating various risk factors that seem to play a role in bringing on the condition.

But what doctors don't understand is why certain people in high risk categories avoid heart attacks and others that avoid all risk categories still suffer heart attacks.

During the past decade, heart researchers have conducted studies on heart attack victims in order to find out what habits these victims have in common. A survey conducted at the Kaiser Permanente Medical Center in Oakland, California, showed that of 464 heart attack victims, a disproportionately high number of the victims had been nondrinkers. After further research, the center revealed that the risk of heart attacks among nondrinkers is 30 percent higher than the risk among moderate drinkers.

The relationship between alcohol consumption and heart attacks has attracted much interest during the past few years. In a recent study comprising all age groups, conducted by the National Institute on Alcohol Abuse and Alcoholism, it was noted that a lower rate of heart attack has been recorded among moderate drinkers than among either heavy drinkers, ex-drinkers, or abstainers.

ALCOHOL AND CHOLESTEROL

Recent studies have revealed that an important relationship exists between a fatty substance called high-density lipo proteins (HDL) and alcohol. People with high HDL levels run a lower risk of heart attacks than people with low HDL levels. HDL is a form of cholesterol, one of the main suspected causes of heart disease. HDL is a different form of cholesterol that scrapes off the fat buildup within the arteries instead of clinging to the walls. A recent study in England showed that moderate to heavy drinkers have a higher level of protective HDL in their blood than nondrinkers. It is reasonable to conclude that the intake of alcohol causes the body to produce additional levels of HDL, which seems to counteract the negative effects of other cholesterol forms in the blood.

ANGINA PECTORIS

Wine has been used since the eighteenth century for the relief of anginal pain. An angina pectoris attack consists of irregular spasms of the coronary arteries that produce stabbing chest pains accompanied by a feeling of suffocation. During an attack, prompt relief of pain is essential.

Wine has been successfully used in treating angina pectoris attacks and diminishing the frequency of subsequent attacks. Many anginal patients find that a breakfast of fruit, lean meat, and tea laced with sherry is a better start for the day than Librium, coffee with cream, eggs and bacon.

Wine consumption, especially brandy, during such attacks, reduces anxiety and controls the severity of the heart pain. The mechanism of this effect is not totally understood, but researchers feel that the relief of pain with alcoholic beverages is somehow mediated through the central nervous system.

The ideal alcoholic therapeutic agent for relief of anginal pain is brandy, which is distilled wine. Beverages with a high alcoholic content are important in order to produce rapid alcohol absorption and a high blood-alcohol peak which allows immediate pain relief. Two ounces of brandy provide sufficient alcohol and ethers to be absorbed directly into the blood, bringing relief of pain within several minutes. Many doctors rate brandy second only to morphine and nitrates in controlling attacks of angina pectoris.

Controlling the fear of paralyzing anginal pain is of primary concern in follow-up therapy. Therefore, many doctors recommend one to two glasses of wine with meals and a glass of port before bed. In selecting wines for the anginal patient, the mineral breakdown of the wine is very important. As an emergency measure to relieve attacks, two ounces of brandy, whiskey, or rum will produce relief of anginal pain within several minutes. As a preventive approach, one to two glasses of either Champagne, sec or brut, or a Médoc with each meal is recommended. Both wines are very high in potassium bitartrate which is important for good muscle tension and coordination, and helps strengthen the heartbeat, providing better oxygenation of the heart.

ARTERIOSCLEROSIS (HARDENING OF THE ARTERIES)

The heart needs a constant supply of blood to stay alive. Arteriosclerosis, the thickening of the artery walls, is a disease of our times, and the most common cause of death in men over forty. Wine can be effectively used to keep the arteries open and free of premature aging and disease. Wine has the ability to dilate the blood vessels, especially the small vessels of the skin. This special aspect of wine can be applied as both a preventive and a curative.

There is strong medical evidence that the addition of wine during meals on a daily basis may reduce the incidence of arteriosclerotic disease by almost 50 percent. It is interesting that wine (as opposed to other alcoholic beverages) when taken with a meal results in lower long-range cholesterol levels than when meals are taken without it. Wine helps soothe the tensions of the day, enabling the diner to relax, enjoying the meal at a much slower tempo. The alcohol in wine, when taken with a meal, is absorbed slowly, and aids in the proper metabolizing of the food. The reduction in the anxiety level alone will moderate the usual hectic pace people set for themselves today. Psychologist Carl Thoreson has stressed the connection between behavior and heart disease, and feels that before stress disorders can be prevented, we must learn how to relax.

Experiments reveal that wine may not only protect against excessive amounts of cholesterol in the arteries, but actually reduce existing deposits. When wine is added to the normal diet, very low levels of cholesterol are accumulated in the blood vessels, even if food high in fat content is consumed.

Roseto, Pennsylvania, has been called the "Miracle Town." For more than eighty years, no person under forty-seven had ever suffered a heart attack. The men worked hard in the local slate quarry, the women took care of the home in an old-world style, and the children were raised in the traditional Italian manner. Meals were family affairs, with ample wine, fatty foods, a diet high in cholesterol. Despite their life-style, the death rate was remarkably low. The incidence of heart disease was one-third the national average.

By 1971, Roseto had become modernized. Dr. John G. Bruhn of the University of Texas, who had initially studied the town ten years earlier, was astounded. Gone were the family dinners, the relaxed atmosphere, the daily consumption of wine. They had been replaced by fast foods, television, and quick beers. The heart disease rate had climbed to the national average.

Both rosé and Muscadet wines are excellent in a preventive approach against arteriosclerosis. The Muscadet vines grow in a soil naturally low in calcium. The low calcium content of Muscadet is extremely important in reducing cholesterol levels. Rosé wines act as mild diuretics and detoxifying agents. Two glasses of wine at meals, alternating daily between a Muscadet and a rosé, is highly recommended.

HYPERTENSION (HIGH BLOOD PRESSURE)

One-third of the U.S. population over fifty is afflicted with hypertension. The body reacts to stress by constricting the artery walls, which raises the blood pressure in the arteries. When the stress situation passes, the blood pressure usually drops back to normal; but if the stress is continual, blood pressure can remain abnormally high.

Medical research has found that alcohol, especially wine, can provide long-lasting relief from the apprehension and general discomfort associated with high blood pressure. Two glasses of wine with meals can reduce the blood pressure for up to four hours. It is not fully understood how the alcohol relieves the symptoms, but most doctors feel the blood pressure is lowered by vascular relaxation as the alcohol works directly on the central nervous system, producing a calming and relaxing effect.

Wine also helps make the normal salt-free diet prescribed for high blood pressure patients more enjoyable. Patients seem to tolerate the diet more readily while learning to relax at mealtime. Relaxation is an extremely important part of re-educating the hypertensive individual.

Light, very dry white wines, with low alcohol levels are highly recommended. These wines have a diuretic effect that promotes the elimination of salt, urine, and uric acid. It is very important for the proper regulation of blood pressure to keep both anxiety and the elimination of unnecessary organic products under control.

HYPOTENSION (LOW BLOOD PRESSURE)

The effects vary greatly, depending on the amount the blood pressure is lowered. Symptoms can range from only momentary giddiness to outright fainting. In a study at the University of California, researchers tested compounds isolated from a California Zinfandel that showed the lower aldehydes of the wine had a definite stimulating effect on blood pressure. Red Burgundy wines that are rich in potassium are extremely beneficial to the nervous and muscular systems. Two to three glasses of wine at meals is recommended.

SORE MUSCLES

Sportsmedicine is the newest prescribed specialty. Joggers, swimmers, tennis players, skiers, and skaters all can be incapacitated by a simple pulled muscle. Karl Jargen, the famous Swedish trainer, developed the following liniment to help relieve lameness quickly:

JOGGER'S LINIMENT

1	egg yolk
1 tablespoon	white wine
1 tablespoon	cider vinegar
1 tablespoon	turpentine

1. Combine all ingredients in a jar.
2. Shake vigorously for several minutes.
   - Rub well into the strained muscle skin surface. Repeat as necessary.

MUSCLE SPASMS

A hot poultice of hops and red wine is extremely effective in relieving muscle cramps. Make the poultice with equal amounts of hops and red wine and apply to affected area.

IMPETIGO

Mothers are undoubtedly familiar with the characteristic crusted-over sores of impetigo known as the "catchingest disease" in the world.

Impetigo is most common between the ages of one and ten, but no age group is exempt. The disease can be transmitted from the slightest touch or infected towel or clothing. Prompt treatment of impetigo is extremely important for a quick and effective cure. If the patient keeps his hands off the infected sores, impetigo can be isolated and controlled within several days.

SWISS IMPETIGO REMEDY

In a glass jar combine equal parts of an acidic red wine and apple cider vinegar. Add 1 teaspoon of sugar per quart of liquid and let stand for 2 hours. Apply directly to lesions 6 to 8 times daily. The impetigo should have disappeared in 2 to 4 days.

If there is no noticeable improvement or the lesions are spreading, see your physician as the infection may be spreading to deeper tissues.

LIVER DISORDERS

Many false ideas concerning wine and the health of the liver have been brought up in recent years by both the medical and nonmedical communities.

Medical research shows that wine, when taken in reasonable amounts, is not dangerous to a healthy liver. In fact, one bottle of wine per day (70 to 80 grams of alcohol) is not considered a health risk in connection with liver function. You would have to drink two and a half times this amount (or 160 to 200 grams) regularly for about twenty-five years to suffer liver damage.

The liver is the primary organ responsible for the metabolism of alcohol. This is accomplished by the secretion of the enzyme *dehydrogenase*, which medical historians have found extremely interesting. Dehydrogenase's only function in the body is to act as a catalyst in alcohol removal, but the enzyme is suspected of being present in the bodies of man's evolutionary ancestors, suggesting the presence of alcohol in the diet since the Stone Age. Alcohol fermentation has been happening naturally for 200 million years, and for better or worse is firmly established into our social structure.

Cirrhosis of the liver is caused by the development of fibrous tissues with consequent scarring, hardening, and the eventual loss of function. Medical research shows that cirrhosis may be caused by malnutrition associated with significant vitamin and protein deficiencies. Unfortunately, cirrhosis of the liver in heavy drinkers has been established, and leads many people to believe falsely that the consumption of alcoholic beverages is the primary cause. Usually alcoholic cirrhosis develops slowly only after many years of alcohol misuse. In fact, many alcoholics never suffer from cirrhosis of the liver while confirmed abstainers develop the condition. As all the data is not as yet complete, the one question that is most important is whether a well-nourished person who "overindulges" is susceptible to cirrhosis. But here we deal again with the question of quantity. The incidence of cirrhosis differs in each country and seems to be influenced by nutritional factors and customs of consumption.

Many major American medical centers have begun to experiment with wine in the treatment of cirrhosis. A test group of alcoholics suffering from cirrhosis, malnutrition, loss of appetite, convulsions, and delirium tremens were started on a high-vitamin and protein diet that included wine, often as much as one liter of dry red wine per day. The group that received the wine responded visibly faster, were more relaxed, and had better appetites. The nutritional approach to treating cirrhosis is vital to improve the function of the liver as well as relieving convulsions. These results only reinforce the importance of the positive effects of wine when consumed in connection with proper nutrition. Wine is actually beneficial to the liver because it is suspected of preventing fatty infiltration by dissipating cholesterol.

THE MENOPAUSE

The menopause is woman's toughest physical and psychological challenge. Her hormonal imbalance causes increased physical stress that many women feel unable or unwilling to accept.

Unfortunately, the menopause coincides with middle age. Women have been taught throughout their lives to attach too much importance to youth. Youthfulness has been associated with sexual attractiveness, the menopause with old age. Therefore, many underlying problems—emotional, psychological, and sexual—come to the surface during this period, and are blamed on "the change."

Some of the more common complaints, such as anxiety, headaches, heart palpitations, tingling, insomnia, nervousness, irritation, and depression, can be treated by a number of methods. During the past few years, estrogen replacement therapy has come under severe attack, and many physicians have switched to the temporary use of tranquilizers and mild sedatives to relieve mild menopausal symptoms.

Dry red wines, especially from the Médoc region of France, have been used successfully throughout Europe in connection with a low-calorie diet to help relieve the symptoms. A California Napa Cabernet is also highly recommended. Many women tend to gain weight during the menopause, which complicates treatment. Two glasses of wine with meals allow the body to relax and adjust to the change.

Many women, especially during menopause, experience frustrating night sweats. To relieve this unpleasant symptom, try the following remedy:

SAGE WINE TEA

Make a strong sage tea, using the herb just as you would any tea. Add 2 tablespoons of red wine for each cup of tea. Drink 3 to 4 cups per day.

MENSTRUAL PROBLEMS

PREMENSTRUAL TENSION

Do you become irritable, tense, nervous? Does your personality change five to ten days before your period? Are you sullen, withdrawn, weepy? Then you suffer from premenstrual tension.

Every woman suffers to a different extent during her monthly cycle, depending on her personality type. The majority of women suffer mild irritating symptoms, but a few women have difficulty coping with the premenstrual phase and its emotional upheavals.

Fortunately, severe problems are in the minority, but that is not to say that women do not suffer from premenstrual tension and related symptoms.

The majority of women complain most about the uncomfortable bloated feeling that occurs during the week preceding menstruation. It is not uncommon for many women to gain as much as five pounds of fluid, causing puffy bloated stomachs, enlarged tender breasts, and bloated feet. Fortunately, this extra fluid is only temporary, but nonetheless, painful.

Although doctors disagree about the exact cause of premenstrual tension, many do see the importance played by water retention, but more importantly, in relief caused by elimination.

Keeping to a low sodium diet is important, but hiding the saltshaker is not enough in today's prepared food paradise. Low-salt meals are a cook's nightmare. So many women turn to an easier answer: the diuretic, or "water pill."

Although synthetic diuretics may improve your disposition, make you easier to live with, and slimmer, they are rarely the right answer. Much of premenstrual tension resulting from monthly hormonal changes stem from emotional instability. But what is the answer?

Many doctors prescribe mild tranquilizers to be taken the week before your period, but despite their effectiveness, the cumulative effect of tranquilizers is widely known.

Fortunately, wine is nature's own tranquilizer and a natural diuretic. Dry white wines are especially helpful in relieving premenstrual tensions. They are low in sodium, but naturally high in potassium. Excessive potassium loss is always considered a problem for women who use synthetic diuretics. Potassium is one of the body's most important elements; a deficiency can cause constipation, intestinal distention, and muscle weakness.

MENSTRUAL CRAMPS

More than half of the female population between the ages of fourteen and forty-five suffer from painful menstruation. The pain usually begins on the first day and lasts about twelve to twenty-four hours. Many women suffer severe disabling cramping during this period. For quick, soothing, symptomatic relief try the following:

CHAMOMILE AND WINE TEA

In a cup soak a chamomile tea bag in 2 tablespoons of strong red Burgundy wine. Add boiling water and let steep for several minutes. Drink 2 to 3 cups of the tea during a 1-hour period.

IRREGULAR MENSTRUAL FLOW

Several years ago I had the pleasure of talking with an Indian medicine chief. He was very knowledgeable on roots and herbs as medicinal preparations. He introduced me to a very interesting medicine called Squaw's Drops, which help regulate menstrual flow or aid in overcoming sluggish painful menstruation.

SQUAW'S DROPS

Prepare a tincture by crushing enough black cohash to half fill a quart bottle. Add equal amounts of whiskey and strong red wine until full. Cover tightly and let stand for 2 weeks. Shake well twice daily. One week before the menstrual period should begin take 5 to 10 drops of mixture in a glass of water 4 times daily. The total daily dose should never exceed 30 drops.

BAD BREATH

Bad breath is a result of poor diet and bad dental hygiene. An interesting mouthwash that will tighten loose gums and freshen the breath comes from Russia. Myrrh is an ancient perfume ingredient that is still used not only in cosmetics but medicinal preparations, and can be purchased at most health food stores.

MYRRH MOUTHWASH

1 cup	100-proof vodka
1/4 cup	strong red wine
2 oz.	powdered myrrh
oil of clove (optional)	

1. Combine all ingredients.
2. Store in a covered jar in a dark place for 2 weeks. Shake daily.
3. Strain into clean container.
4. Add oil of clove if desired for aroma.
 • Use as often as necessary.

The French use a light, fresh white or rosé wine swished around in the mouth. Wine acts as an excellent cleansing, astringent mouthwash.

For variety in your mouthwash, try infusing different herbs in white wine. Take a handful of clove, myrrh, licorice, peppermint, or spearmint and add to a bottle of dry white wine. Set aside for ten days. I like the spearmint in a dry Chablis—it's especially nice.

A dentist in Rome recommended the following preparation to strengthen gums and help tighten loose teeth: Dissolve one ounce of myrrh in two cups of strong dry red wine and two cups of oil of almonds. Rinse the mouth every morning.

POISON IVY, POISON OAK

Poison ivy and poison oak need little introduction to nature lovers. The intense itching and skin lesions which follow contact have ruined many vacations. The initial rash usually begins between twelve and forty-eight hours after contact and persists for about two weeks. Unfortunately contact does not have to be direct. Many unsuspecting victims have been infected from pets, clothing, or from smoke from burning plants.

There are many varied approaches to treatment. The best, of course, is to avoid the plant. But if you are too late to prevent the rash entirely, be sure to cleanse the skin thoroughly with a strong soap.

Mountain climbers for generations have used this simple

treatment to help cure skin eruptions and rashes caused by the poisonous plants: Take a very hot shower or bath. The heat of the water will release histamine, which will cause intense itching. Increase the temperature of the water as the itching increases. Continue this procedure until the maximum hot water temperature tolerable is reached. Apply straight dry white wine to the skin; pat dry—do not rub skin. The method should give you at least eight hours of relief from itching. Apply the wine as often as necessary, especially during the night to get some sleep. If a shower or bath is not convenient, try hot compresses.

RINGWORM

During the last several years, the United States has been experiencing a ringworm epidemic. Ringworm is a fungus infection of the skin involving small, locally inflamed reddish patches. The patches may be single or multiple and usually involve the head area. On close investigation, rounded, scaly, bald patches are visible where the hair shafts are broken off close to the scalp.

Although no one is immune, children are more often affected because the fungus can be easily transmitted from child to child by swapping hats or resting the head against high-backed seats in movie theaters. Ringworm should be treated promptly to stop the spread of the lesions. The mixture below is an excellent antiseptic and effective antifungal agent.

RINGWORM REMEDY

In a pan heat 1 cup of red wine and ½ cup of apple cider vinegar. Massage the mixture with your fingers directly into the infected area 6 times a day.

KICK THE SMOKING HABIT IN 14 DAYS

From the Orient comes gentian, a plant that has proved a very successful substitute for tobacco. A gentian tonic is an excellent remedy for anyone interested in breaking themselves of the smoking habit.

GENTIAN TONIC

1 pint	gentian root
1 cup	Burgundy wine
1 cup	water

1. Combine all ingredients.
2. Cover the mixture and let stand 14 days.
   - Take 1 teaspoon 4 times a day for 2 weeks. The desire for tobacco will gradually decrease and eventually be gone.

HOW TO SHRINK VARICOSE VEINS

An old folk medicine remedy from Germany to help shrink varicose veins is still widely prescribed throughout Europe.

Mix equal quantities of dry white wine and apple cider vinegar. Apply with your hand directly to varicose veins twice daily in the morning and before bed at night.

By the end of the first month shrinking of the veins should be visible.

To increase effectiveness, each morning drink an eight-ounce glass of mineral water to which two teaspoons each of apple cider vinegar and dry white wine have been added.

PART TWO

WINE AND YOUR LOOKS

CHAPTER SEVEN

WINE AND YOUR LOOKS

Wine for centuries has been helping people around the world feel and look good.

What is a beautiful woman? Or a handsome, virile man? He or she may not have a stereotyped physique, but they both know how to make the most of their looks. They have a special quality—an inner glow—that makes them beautiful.

After interviewing hundreds of people in ten different countries for this section of the book, I began to realize the importance wine can have in building the separate parts of beauty—smooth complexion, shining hair, healthy white teeth, a sleek figure. Each part of the body has to be cared for and the subtle way in which they are combined creates the youthful, vibrant you.

In the following chapters you can discover dozens of useful wine hints on how to keep your body young, healthy, and attractive. This is not the usual book on makeup and exercise, but an exciting international trip with secret wine cures that will help you make the most of your looks.

CHAPTER EIGHT

THE DRINK YOURSELF
THIN DIET

HOW TO DIET SUCCESSFULLY
WITH WINE!

Losing weight has become a national obsession. More than 40 million Americans went on a diet this year, but less than two percent were successful and permanently maintained their desired weight goal. The most widely asked question I received while researching this book was, Can I drink wine, stay healthy, and still be slim? Happily, the answer is yes!

WEIGHT MAINTENANCE

Calculating how to maintain or achieve your ideal body weight is an important part of dieting with wine. Recognizing and calculating the extra-calorie problem is the first step on a successful reducing program. Understanding and evaluating your daily calorie requirement plus calculating the number of calories you actually consume will help establish a lasting diet program that will be beneficial for you.

How many calories do you need? How many calories do you actually consume? The magic number isn't pulled out of a hat, it is simply calculated by multiplying your body weight by 15. A 130-pound woman needs 1,950 calories daily (or 130 times 15 = 1,950). For the jogger or person who does hard physical labor, the factor of 15 must be increased to 25; therefore, a 180-pound man needs approximately 4,500 calories daily (or 180 times 25 = 4,500) to maintain his body weight.

Americans eat their main meal in the evening, which is the very worst way to diet successfully. Europeans eat most heavily early in the day, which maximizes calorie burn efficiency.

When alcohol is added to the diet, the alcohol is burned for energy and the food is deposited as fat. Therefore, the cocktail party drinker who has three or four with hors d'oeuvres before a large dinner party will undoubtedly suffer from a socially induced weight problem.

The sensible dieter who wants to enjoy wine while dieting will consume high-calorie foods early in the day when the body can best utilize the food for energy. It is very important to insure continued good health that proper nutrition is observed while dieting.

The late afternoon and evening hours are the worst for the dieter. On the Drink-Yourself-Thin Diet, wine is allowed one to two hours before dinner and throughout the evening as long as there is no snacking, because wine calories will be easily burned and are not converted to body fat.* Although wine is allowed, exact calorie count is required. The chart that follows, which I have developed over the past several years, is essential in recording caloric values.

Dieting is a form of self-torture, but the Drink-Yourself-Thin Diet is more a self-improvement program in which the dieter begins to understand his own body. Many people have begun to follow it with enthusiasm and within a few days, wives, husbands, friends, and golfing partners begin watching wide-eyed as the pounds fade away—permanently. The secret is simple, so tighten your belt and throw away the girdles. Estimate your ideal weight and calculate your daily calorie count. No cheating—count *everything*. Begin drinking wine before dinner, stop snacking, and watch the pounds melt away.

*In the body alcohol is converted into acetate and these molecules are then burned by combining with oxygen. If the body is oxygen-deficient, some of the acetate will be converted into fat, but adequate daily doses of vitamins B1, B6, biotin, and E will increase the body's natural oxygen level and avoid fat buildup.

This is not a crash diet; rather it's a slow but sure method of permanent and pleasant weight reduction. Most diets forbid or severely restrict alcohol consumption, but as soon as the diet is finished and you begin drinking again, the lost weight is rapidly regained.

If you have suffered through the hundreds of diets on the market today without lasting success, the Drink-Yourself-Thin Diet is for you. But as with any diet, see your doctor first and never mix wine with other medications without your physician's recommendation.

Dieting with wine is a pleasant gradual weight-loss regimen that usually results in a three-to-five-pound loss per month until the desired permanent weight is reached.

ADDING UP THE CALORIES

"I don't know how I can be overweight—I hardly eat anything!"

Physicians and diet counselors hear this statement countless times by overweight people who diet unsuccessfully. The key to understanding yourself and how you eat is recognizing your daily calorie intake.

"I'm going to start dieting tomorrow!" How many times have you heard someone say it? How many times have you said it yourself? Successful dieting is an art that few people ever achieve, because they make a commitment to a diet, not to themselves!

Tomorrow, start your diet by eating normally—be honest, and using the calorie counter in Appendix B write down the total calories you consume. Then add them up!

Elizabeth is a 135-pound woman who sits at a desk every day and does relatively light exercise on the weekend. Her daily calorie intake is 2,800, but Elizabeth only needs 2,025 calories daily to maintain her 135-pound weight.

The body requires 3,500 calories to gain one pound of fat. Therefore, without any diet modification, Elizabeth will gain a little more than one pound per week.

The diet of the average American is a disaster. More people suffer from overconsumption malnutrition than any other disease. Common sense is the single most important element lacking in our diet.

CALORIC VALUES OF WINES

Wines	Calories per Ounce (Approx.)
Red table wine	18
Dry white table wine	20
Catawba (sweet)	30
Champagne (brut)	21
Champagne (extra dry)	29
Madeira	32
Port (U.S.)	43
Porto (imported)	39
Sherry (U.S.)	36
Sherry (dry, imported)	32
Vermouth (dry, French)	27
Vermouth (sweet, Italian)	44
Liqueurs Bénédictine, Chartreuse, Drambuie, and other generic liqueurs	100–120

Tables of Food Values—Revised and Enlarged by Alice V. Bradley (Pub. Chas. A. Bennett Co., Inc., Peoria, Illinois).

The wine diet eliminates the antisocial stigma of dieting. It's fun and successful. The following comments from satisfied wine dieters attest to its effectiveness.

Sara K. lost thirty-five pounds over a doctor-supervised six-month period. "I was a nervous eater, more a snacker, beginning after work at four o'clock and continuing through until bedtime. Wine helps me relax; one glass satisfies my snacking urges for hours."

Peter W. was ordered by his doctor to lose twenty pounds. "For more than ten years, I had been dieting unsuccessfully. My greatest weakness was an uncontrollable sweet tooth. After one or two glasses of dry wine at dinner, sweets taste awful. Now, if I feel the urge for a candy bar, I pour myself a small glass of dry sherry and sip it slowly. It works every time."

Betty S. lost ten pounds and has succesfully kept them off. "I was a nocturnal refrigerator raider. One glass of wine before bedtime helps me relax and reduces my midnight 'munchy' raids."

Michael P. has finally reached his desired weight after years of fluctuation. "Drinking wine with my dinner has helped me enormously to cut my calorie count. I eat slower and much less while I sip my wine. It has changed my life ... I love it!"

Ralph J., a busy executive, lost twenty pounds. "I was concerned naturally about my ballooning weight, but the amount of alcohol I was drinking—two martinis at lunch, cocktails before dinner, even a beer at bedtime! My wife continually complained about my spare tire. I was miserable. The wine diet not only helped me lose weight, but I enjoy life more— I'm more relaxed. I guess you could say I dine now, not eat."

CHAPTER NINE

NATURAL BEAUTY SECRETS FROM THE VINEYARDS

Everyone wants to look good. Beauty is an elusive quality that women for centuries have fought to maintain against the ravages of time. Throughout history, women have coated their skins with everything from mud to grease. Alchemists have dedicated their lives to concocting complicated formulas that would keep the skin youthful—many were successful, others fatal. In the eighteenth century, women took arsenic to achieve petal-soft white complexions.

Today, many of the most expensive commercial cosmetics contain harmful, even toxic ingredients. It is even doubtful that these products produce the results that the advertisers make us believe we need.

Is there another answer? Throughout my travels around the world, I have been intrigued by women who have enhanced their attractiveness through simple, natural methods. The skin is your personal barometer of health, indicating what is happening throughout your body. Why not listen? The human body responds to special care, as a plant thrives when exposed to sun and water. With a little extra effort, your life can take on a new vitality, a sparkle. You'll have a prettier, healthier body. Your skin will be younger, fresher, glowing, free from everyday tension lines. Even if you are one of the lucky few who are blessed with a naturally beautiful complexion, it still must be nurtured daily to maintain its natural glowing radiance.

Beauty and health are closely related. Your actual physical

beauty is directly derived from good health. Aging is inevitable, but why let the years leave their mark before their time? By actively pursuing a natural beauty regimen, you can gain many beautiful and rewarding years.

The search for beauty is exciting and by no means limited to the few women who can afford expensive cosmetics. With today's organic health trend, more women are questioning the transitory effects of expensive chemically produced cosmetic products. Nature is rich with inexpensive organic beauty supplies. While traveling through Europe, I discovered the important part that wine has played in natural beauty cures for centuries. Even today wine is still the single most common ingredient that I found in all the natural beauty recipes. Rich in vitamins and minerals, wine interacts with specific natural ingredients to help cleanse and beautify the skin, the hair, the entire body.

By following the simple natural beauty secrets included in this book, you can in a relatively short time create an inner health—a vigorous, wholesome beauty that will radiate in your complexion.

For generations, women have known that the skin does not lie. Famous beauties throughout the centuries have relied on secret formulas to retain their youth. The recipes of these concoctions have been jealously guarded. After interviewing women around the world, I have compiled some of their more exciting natural beauty secrets that derive their success directly from wine. I am sure you will feel a tremendous difference from the first applications. You owe it to yourself to be the best you can be. A woman at her best is poised, confident, on top of the world—beautiful.

CARE FOR YOUR SKIN

Cleansing, toning, and nourishing are the three most important requirements of a healthy skin-care program. If daily care is neglected, the skin will suffer.

After the age of twenty-five, the skin loses some of its normal elasticity and extra care should be focused around the sensitive tissue-paper-thin eye area which is especially susceptible to wrinkles. As you grow older, your cells do not rejuvenate themselves as quickly as they did before. It is necessary to aid nature by cleansing and often scrubbing away the dead cells to allow the new growth of cells to breathe. This procedure actually slows down aging and makes you more beautiful. But it is important to select the correct beauty aids. The following cures can help your skin feel smoother, moist, and younger-looking, thus making you more beautiful.

START WITH A CLEAN FACE

For an ancient but still effective cleanser, combine one egg yolk with two teaspoons of almond oil and one teaspoon of white wine. Wash the skin with mixture, rinse, and pat dry.

To clean out your pores, fill a small muslin bag with bran. Put the bag into a small pan filled with boiling white wine for several minutes. Remove and dab your face with the warm wine bag.

FRUIT MASKS

Europeans have been using masks and packs made from a variety of vegetables, fruits, and nuts for centuries. Masks can be applied to any part of the body and are used by as many men as women. They are successful in clearing blackheads or pimples, refining pores and moisturizing, as well as absorbing excess oil, nourishing, soothing, and healing traumatized skin.

The secret and most successful beauty ingredient in masks and packs is wine. Wine helps the individual fruit or vegetable naturally refine and clean out the pores, and tighten sagging flesh. The first step in selecting a mask or pack is to determine your individual skin type.

DRY TO NORMAL SKIN

Apple	Nectarines
Avocado	Oranges
Grapes	Orange Flowers
Honeydew Melon	Pears
Irish Moss	Watermelon

Banana	Cranshaw Melon	Tangerine
Cantaloupe	Casaba Melon	Zucchini
Carrot	Marigold	
Citrus	Peach	
	Peppermint	

OILY SKIN

Apricot leaves	Lemon Grass
Avocado Oil	Persian Melon
Bananas	Peppermint Oil
Cherry	Tomato
Lemons	
Lemon Peel	

BASIC MASK RECIPE

1. Mash the fruit*, taking care to squeeze out all the juice.
2. Add 2–3 tablespoons of dry white wine; let stand for 5 minutes.
  • Apply pulp to face. Lie down with feet raised for 20 minutes. Rinse with cool water. Pat dry.

*The following fruits are recommended for correcting specific skin problems:

1. Apples and pears	Smooth
2. Apricots, peaches, nectarines, melons	Refine and texturize the skin
3. Blueberries, black currants	Protect delicate skin capillaries
4. Grapes and pears	Moisturize skin; rejuvenate facial muscles
5. Lemons, oranges, grapefruits, and all citrus fruits	Tone and clean (antiseptic)

| 6. Strawberries | Reduce oiliness; soften skin |
| 7. Watermelons | Help remove fine line wrinkles |

To refine large pores combine one tablespoon of almond meal with several drops of white wine until it is spreadable. Use like beauty-washing grains, but leave on for 20 minutes. Rinse with warm water.

To soften dry skin add ½ cup of cold milk and ½ cup of white wine to 1 ounce of ground almonds. Mix thoroughly and then strain. Add ½ ounce of sugar. Spread mixture on skin and let stand for twenty minutes. Wash face and hands with warm water.

To tone oily skin, apples have been used for centuries. Grate a large apple into a dish and add 2 tablespoons of white wine. Spread mixture over face while lying down on a towel. Leave on for 20 minutes, then wash with warm water.

To soothe dry skin, try this treatment from the Pennsylvania Dutch country. Slice an apple in ½-inch wedges and scratch the surface with a serrated knife. Soak the slices in fermented apple cider or a very dry white wine for 5 minutes. Lie down. Rub the apple slices across the entire surface of your skin and let set for 20–30 minutes. Rinse with warm water (no soap) and rub on a thin layer of nut oil. You should see an immediate improvement in your complexion.

From Buenos Aires comes this wonderful avocado facial mask. In a blender mash one avocado with one teaspoon of white wine and an egg white. Apply to face; wait 25 minutes. Wash with warm water. An excellent cure for dry tired skin.

From England comes a facial mask that will not only cleanse deeply but improve circulation. Mix enough powdered barley with 2 teaspoons of white wine until a paste is formed. More wine may be needed to achieve the correct consistency. Smooth on skin, let dry, then wash with warm water.

Many Swiss skin specialists recommend carrots for a weekly youthful facial. Carrots are rich in vitamins that are effective both inside and out for beauty treatments. Cook about 5 large carrots until soft; drain water. Add 2 tablespoons of white wine. Let stand for 10 minutes. Mix into smooth paste. Apply to face; wait 30 minutes. Wash with warm water.

In Holland women soothe tired skin after removing their makeup by rubbing their faces with a slice of cucumber that has been soaked in a dry white wine. It has a cleansing, cooling effect. In England the same application is used to counter oily skin by mashing the cucumber, sprinkling on the wine, and letting it set all day.

The cool, tingly cucumber mask is rich in natural silicon and sulphur, and its application as a beauty product throughout the world has intrigued me. Try the following mask from Switzerland:

SWISS CUCUMBER MASK

½ cup	chopped cucumber
2 tablespoons	dry white wine
2 teaspoons	powdered milk
1	egg white

1. In a blender combine the cucumber and wine; let stand for 3 minutes.
2. Add the powdered milk and egg white.
3. Blend into a smooth paste.
   - Apply with swirling motions to face and neck. Allow the mask to dry for approximately 30 minutes. Rinse with warm water first, then rinse again with cool water and blot dry.

The dandelion is an excellent source of the beauty vitamins A, B, C, and G as well as iron, calcium, potassium, magnesium, and silicon. An infusion of dandelions makes an indispensable face wash that can help strengthen facial muscles while cleansing tissues and alleviating sallowness.

DANDELION FACIAL PACK

1 cup	minced dandelion leaves
1½ cups	cold water
¼ cup	dry white wine

1. In a saucepan combine the minced dandelion leaves, water, and wine.
2. Slowly bring the mixture to a boil; simmer for 15 minutes.
3. Remove from heat and cool.
   - Lie down, elevate your feet, and with a sterile gauze wipe the mixture over your entire face. Soak two large pads in the mixture and place them on each cheek for 20 minutes. Rinse with warm water, then cool water, and pat dry. Continue the facial 3 times a week for 4–6 weeks. A noticeable improvement should be observed within 2 weeks. The facial should be prepared from fresh dandelion leaves. Don't run to the health food store; try your lawn, garden, or nearest park.

THE GRAPE FACIAL

Green grapes contain less iron than their purple cousins, but in the Rhineland they are considered the perfect restorative facial for tired summer skin. Nothing compares to the richness of the grape harvest. In Italy, iron-rich red grapes have been considered a beauty potion for centuries. In September, when the grapes are at their best, mash ½ pound of grapes and add three tablespoons of red wine. Let the mixture stand for 1 hour and apply to both face and neck areas. The combined action of the wine and the alkaline grape, rich in potassium, sulphur, and phosphorus plus vitamins A, B, and C, will help relieve many skin disorders as well as cleansing and strengthening the skin.

HONEY MASKS

Most masks are more successful when applied to a freshly steamed, clean face. First apply a small slightly wrung out hot towel to your face, lie down with feet elevated so the blood rushes to the face for ten minutes. Try 3 egg whites, whipped with 1 tablespoon of red wine and 1 tablespoon of honey. When applied to the face in a rotating motion, the mask stimulates and refines enlarged pores.

HONEY-WINE PAT

Honey is a natural rejuvenator, hydrator, and a cosmetic miracle. Skin ages not because it has lost the ability to retain oil, but because it loses water. The Honey-Wine Pat leaves the skin tight and firm, and due to its acid content helps rid the face of blackheads and pimples.

Take ¼ cup of honey and heat together with 3 tablespoons of red wine. Heat over low heat until warm. Pat the mixture on your face and neck with your fingertips. Relax. Let set for 10 minutes. Rinse with tepid water.

There are a great variety of honey-wine facials that can be used every day to moisturize, invigorate, soften, and help alleviate these fine wrinkling lines that develop on the face:

- Anemic skin can benefit enormously from honey, which stimulates and nourishes fatigued skin. Make a mask by beating together 1 teaspoon of honey and 1 teaspoon of red wine.
- For relief of oily skin, mix ½ teaspoon of honey with 1 tablespoon of white wine. Combine with enough powdered barley to achieve spreading consistency. More wine may be added if needed.

Try the following honey wine masks:

Skin Type	Mask Preparation
Normal/oily	1 teaspoon honey, 1 teaspoon white wine, 1 teaspoon mashed banana
Dry/normal	1 teaspoon honey, 1 teaspoon rosé wine, 1 teaspoon unbeaten egg white
Colorless	1 teaspoon honey, 1 teaspoon red wine, 1 teaspoon orange juice

| Dry/flaky | 1 teaspoon honey, 1 teaspoon white wine, ½ teaspoon egg yolk |
| Dry | 1 teaspoon honey, 1 teaspoon white wine, ½ teaspoon corn oil. |

In Sweden honey plays a major part in many beauty treatments.

To soften dry skin, try this recipe:

HONEY-EGG-WINE MASK

½ teaspoon	honey
1	egg yolk
1 tablespoon	white wine
1–2 tablespoons	dry skim milk

1. Combine all ingredients.
2. Stir until paste is formed.
   • Apply to face and neck;
     wait for 20 minutes. Rinse with warm water.

SMOOTHERS, LIGHTENERS, AND BERRY BEAUTIFIERS

Have you ever envied the beautiful clear complexions of the Irish colleens? How are they able to maintain such creamy, soft skins in the harsh Irish climate?

It is important to nourish the skin, and Irish beauties have known the secrets of the potato for centuries. When the common potato is added to your daily beauty regimen your skin is bathed in vitamins B, C, and G, and sulphur, and takes on a soft, supple appearance. If used daily, the cure will improve oily skin without developing the small dry lines around the mouth and eyes that very often appear with commercially prepared products.

POTATO OILY SKIN CURE

1 medium-sized potato
dry white wine

1. Cut potato in half.
2. With a serrated knife, crisscross the potato until the center becomes pulpy.
3. Stand potato on cut side in saucer of wine for 30 minutes.
   - Rub cut side of potato over your face for 1–2 minutes, allowing the liquid to dry on your skin for approximately 20 minutes. Rinse with clear cold water and pat dry.

Brewer's yeast is an important beauty food that should be included in any smart beauty plan. Rich in vitamin B, amino acids, and minerals, brewer's yeast is a high protein product that can help create a rosy, glowing complexion. Most nutritionists feel that for best results, brewer's yeast should be taken internally as well as applied as a mask. The recommended dosage is one teaspoon daily dissolved in fruit juice at first, working up to a final dosage of three tablespoons daily. The following mask stimulates the skin, smoothing out wrinkles and facial lines.

YEAST MASK

1 tablespoon	powdered brewer's yeast
3 tablespoons	milk
1 tablespoon	white wine

1. Mix together all ingredients to form a paste.
   - Apply to a warm clean face and neck. Let dry 20–30 minutes. Loosen with hot face cloth dipped into warm water that has two tablespoons of white wine added. Massage the face with the warm water until all traces of the mask are gone. (If dryness develops, apply a thin layer of cream or oil around eyes and throat area.)

As summer turns to fall those lovely tans begin to yellow, leaving the complexion sallow, and a suntan bleach may be needed. French beauties for centuries have relied on the following cures to remove their leftover tan.

CRANBERRY LIGHTENER

The cranberry contains four important acids that help bleach skin. If you find the application too astringent, shorten the period of use.

1 lb.	fresh cranberries
4 tablespoons	red wine

1. Crush cranberries and extract the juice.
2. Mix in wine.
3. Pour into a glass container and refrigerate when not in use.
   - Apply the juice mixture to the face and neck and other parts of the body. The juice may be left on overnight and rinsed off in the morning with cool water. The bleaching process may take several days until the complexion is lighter and rosier.

LEMON-WINE FACIAL CREAM

1	lemon
½ cup	whole milk
3 tablespoons	white wine
yogurt	

1. Combine milk and wine.
2. Slice lemon and soak for several hours in milk mixture.
3. Remove lemon and add enough yogurt to milk mixture to thicken.
   - Gently rub the cream into your face and let sit for 1–2 hours. Rinse with warm water. Pat dry.

STRAWBERRY CREAM FACIAL MASK

The strawberry mask is extremely effective in lightening and softening the skin. It is especially effective on deeply tanned complexions that have taken on a yellow tinge.

1 pt.	strawberries
2 tablespoons	red wime
1 pt.	heavy cream

1. Mash strawberries in a wooden bowl.
2. Add wine and let stand for 10 minutes.
3. Add cream and stir.
   - Apply mixture to face and throat. Wait 30 minutes, then rinse off with cool water and pat dry.

PEACHES AND CREAM MASK

For a truly English peaches-and-cream complexion with that special blushing glow try this:

1	very ripe peach
2 tablespoons	white wine
3 tablespoons	heavy cream

1. Slice peach and mash.
2. Sprinkle peach with wine and let stand for 1 hour.
3. Add cream and mix.
   - Massage the mask into your skin and wait 20 minutes, then rinse off with cool water and pat dry.

ACNE

Acne is a superficial skin eruption that is a frequent problem in adolescents with oily skin. The most effective preventive approach is cleanliness, but grease and creams may aggravate the condition. (Diet alone is usually not the determining factor.) Most over-the-counter products help some cases and are disappointing in others. Acne attacks are not only physically but emotionally painful, and emergency measures are very often needed. If you have a teenager in tears caused by severe facial eruptions, try the following treatments:

PAPAYA FACIAL

2	papaya mint tea bags
1½ cups	water
2 tablespoons	red wine

1. Add wine to water and bring to boil.
2. Steep the tea bags in the hot water and wine mixture.
3. Keep the liquid as hot as can be tolerated.
   - Saturate a cloth and apply to face for 20 minutes, reheating cloth as it cools. Repeat procedure twice daily. A noticeable improvement should be seen within several hours; within several days the eruptions should have disappeared.

ALOE-ALMOND-WINE MASK

1	aloe plant
1 teaspoon	almond meal
1 tablespoon	cold-pressed oil
1½ teaspoons	rosé wine

1. Take the inner pulp from an aloe plant (approximately 2 well-rounded tablespoons) and combine with the almond meal and wine.
2. Let stand for 2 minutes.
3. Add the oil and form the ingredients into a gooey meal.
   - Apply to skin using upward rotating motions. Relax and let the mixture stay on for 15 minutes, then rinse with warm water. Follow the facial with an astringent.

AUSTRIAN ACNE MASK

The three ingredients of this mask are carrots, yogurt, and white wine. Carrots are rich in vitamin A, which helps build a natural resistance to infection, but when used externally helps clear up pimples and especially acne. Yogurt promotes the growth of helpful bacteria and used on the skin provides calcium and protein. When wine is added to these two ingredients, it helps activate their natural healing properties faster to bring much-needed relief.

1	raw carrot
2 tablespoons	plain natural yogurt
1 tablespoon	rosé wine

1. In a blender combine all ingredients until well mixed.
   - Apply the mixture to your skin in light upward rotating movements. Let it stay on for 15 minutes and wash off with cool *mineral* water.

BLACKHEADS

These tiny little black pits that plague so many complexions are the focal point of almost fifty different beauty products found on today's market.

Blackheads can be removed by several methods: Herbal steams, beauty grains, or hot compresses.

Beauty grains are a terrific blackhead scrub. Try oatmeal, cornmeal, or almond meal slightly moistened with white wine several times a week. (Cornmeal mixed with white wine is especially cleansing.)

Try the following hot compresses for a clearer complexion:
- Mash an apricot in honey. Add enough red wine to cover. Heat for 10 minutes on a low flame. Apply mixture to blackhead area.
- Soak several tansy leaves (available in all health food stores) in 3 tablespoons of white wine and buttermilk for several hours. Strain the liquid and warm; apply as often as necessary.

BLEMISH TEA

½ oz.	comfrey leaf
1 oz.	burdock root
½ oz.	sassafras root
½ oz.	red clover
½ oz.	dandelion leaf
1 oz.	violet leaves and flowers
1 cup	boiling water
½ cup	white wine

1. Combine all the herbs in a pan.
2. Add the water and the white wine.
3. Strain.
   - Drink throughout the day, as well as apply as a warm compress.

Special Note: All the herbal ingredients may be found at health food stores.

FACIAL PEELING

Facial peeling can be easily done at home. After the outer layer of skin is removed, your skin should be rosy and shining.

The French use a variety of fruits as peeling agents; pineapple, lime, tomato, or lemon are extremely effective. The face should be steamed clean before beginning the peeling procedure.

FRUIT FACIAL PEEL

Fresh fruit
3 tablespoons white wine

1. Mash the fruit into a pulp including any fresh juice from the skin.
2. Add wine.
3. Let stand for 1 hour.
4. Drain.
   - Apply the drained fruit pulp to your face in smooth, circular motions. Rinse with warm water first, then cool. Pat dry.

On the Riviera I was introduced to an avocado oil rejuvenator. It is a facial peel that I will always remember, and I indulge myself once a month.

AVOCADO OIL REJUVENATOR

Massage 1 teaspoon avocado oil combined with 1 teaspoon white wine into your skin with circular motions for 5–10 minutes. Either almond or a germ oil may be substituted for the avocado oil.

DEVON RUB

For a truly beautiful English peaches-and-cream complexion:

Combine 1 teaspoon peppermint water and 1 teaspoon white wine. Rub this mixture into your skin with circular motions. After 30 seconds, you should begin to feel a small ball develop, but keep rubbing until your entire face feels smooth and wonderful. This massage is very effective after weeks of drying summer sun.

DRY, TIRED SKIN

Dry, tired skin plagues everyone at some time of the year. Prolonged exposure to the harsh winter winds or drying summer sun can make any complexion dull and lifeless. A nutritional, reviving facial can do much to restore vitality to your complexion.

Salon facials can be prohibitively expensive, but the following rich creamy natural facial, used daily, will return your skin to its smooth, silky, lineless beauty for less than a penny a day. The protein-based facial slowly feeds the tissues and softens damaged skin. After a thirty-minute application, the facial tissues will be noticeably firmer.

MIRACLE TISSUE CREAM

1 egg	
2 tablespoons	dry white wine
½ teaspoon	salt
1 cup	cold processed salad oil
4 tablespoons	collagenous protein (can be bought at any health food store)
4 tablespoons	oatmeal water (see below)

1. In a blender mix the egg, wine, salt, and ½ cup of the salad oil at high speed until slightly thickened.
2. Remove the blender cover and pour in the remaining oil while still blending. This makes the basic cream.
3. To the cream, add the collagenous protein and the oatmeal water. Beat well.
4. Keep refrigerated until needed.

BASIC OATMEAL WATER

1. Soak 2 tablespoons of oatmeal in 6 tablespoons of hot water for 10 minutes and 2 tablespoons of white wine.
2. Strain mixture and reserve milky fluid.

HERBAL WINE STEAM FACIAL

The basic herbal steam facial is the standard cure for dry, flaking skin. Each application helps remove the top layer of dead skin allowing a glowing fresh porcelain-textured healthy new underskin to appear.

2	papaya mint tea bags
2 cups	boiling water
½ cup	white wine

1. Combine all ingredients.
2. Simmer for 5 minutes.
   - The mixture should be used very warm because the interaction between the heat and the herbal mixture loosens the dead skin.

Timing is extremely important in steam facials. Moist, hot cloths that have been soaked in the herbal mixture must be applied to the face for 15–20 minutes for a successful application. When the cloths cool, the procedure is repeated.
After the facial, rinse your face with cool water and apply a thin layer of fruit oil. For best effects, the herbal facial should be applied in the evening, before retiring.

PAPAYA RUB

If your problem is broken facial veins, avoid very hot compresses and apply the Papaya Rub:

Mash a very ripe papaya in a small glass dish with enough red wine to make a paste. Spread the mixture on your face for 30 minutes and rinse with warm water. Rub the warm skin gently with your fingertips for 2 minutes, rinse again with warm water, then cool. Pat dry.

SWEDISH SKIN REFRESHER

Swedish athletes have relied on this simple cure for years to relieve dry, flaky winter skin. There is no need anymore to suffer from that dull gray winter look. With only a few minutes every week, you can have a healthy glow to your complexion despite the season.

Distilled water	
1 teaspoon	salt
1 teaspoon	white wine

1. Fill a small spray bottle with distilled water.
2. Dissolve salt in wine and add to water.
   - With your eyes and mouth closed, spray a light layer of the solution over your face and neck area. Allow to dry about 1 minute. There should be a tight feeling. Then in circular movements with your fingers, rub the entire facial area gently. The friction will remove the dead, useless cellular top skin. The undersurface should be glowing. Rinse well several times with cool water and apply your favorite cream.

Next we travel to the Caribbean for a simple and effective nourishing skin cream.

CRÉME HAITI

Combine 2 ounces of coconut oil, 1½ fluid ounces of elderflower water, 2½ fluid ounces of rose water, 2 ounces of lanolin, and 2 ounces of white wine.

CUCUMBER COOLER

Cucumber juice is a cooling natural astringent and when combined with wine makes an excellent natural beauty treatment.
- To cool sunburns combine equal amounts of cucumber juice with white wine.
- For a quick pick-me-up for an oily nose, soak a cotton pad in the same solution as above.

CUCUMBER PICK-ME-UP

The summer sun and heat increases the oil production of the skin. For a fresher, more supple complexion, refresh your skin several times daily with the Cucumber Pick-Me-Up:

1	chopped cucumber
1 teaspoon	witch hazel
1 teaspoon	white wine

1. Peel and chop the cucumber.
2. Reduce to pulp in blender and extract all the juice.
3. Combine cucumber juice, witch hazel, and wine in a glass container. Keep refrigerated.
   • Wipe the skin to cleanse several times daily.

FACE FRESHENER

Champagne and sparkling mineral water combine to make a nice Face Freshener. This is especially refreshing after jogging or several sets of tennis.

Fill a plant mister or small atomizer bottle with a sparkling mineral water—try Vichy, Evian, or Perrier. For each quart of water, add ½ cup of dry Champagne. It will leave you with a fresh, tingling complexion.

SHAVING SAVERS

Men have fewer wrinkles. Did you ever wonder why? The answer is simple: they shave them off daily. Shaving removes the dead outer layer of skin, but this daily assault to the facial tissues can be irritating. To maintain a clear, smooth, youthful skin you need to apply a soothing tonic at least three times per week.

THE SKIN SAVER

2 ounces	witch hazel extract
2 ounces	mucilage of quince (available at health food stores)
2 tablespoons	red wine
2–3 drops	lemon oil

Mix together and splash on after shaving to help soothe irritated underskin.

Here is another treatment for skin irritated by daily shaving. Take equal parts of apricot pulp and honey; mix together with 1 part red wine. Apply in the shower or after a steam pack, when the heat will help the honey penetrate.

WRINKLES

Since the beginning of time women have tried to elude wrinkles and facial lines. Multi-billion dollar empires have been established in the cosmetics industry to help society cheat the aging process. Both men and women feel any attempt to avoid the appearance of aging and evade the inevitable wrinkle is worthwhile. Wrinkled, leathery skin makes anybody look old before their time. Today, with the increased interest in jogging, more people are experiencing complexion problems related to continual exposure to the weather.

Many doctors feel that a protein deficiency can cause premature wrinkling. If you are on an extended reducing diet, plan to feed your skin liberally with a protein lotion to help avoid weight-loss wrinkles.

Egyptian women relied on egg whites beaten with several drops of white wine. The mixture was patted on the skin, allowed to dry for thirty minutes then rinsed with warm water.

Austrian women have found that a puréed banana mixed with three tablespoons of white wine helps relieve skin tightness that leads to wrinkling.

Danish beauties follow this simple facial daily to avoid wrinkling. Combine one tablespoon oatmeal, three or four drops each of salad oil and heavy cream, and one teaspoon white wine. Massage this mixture gently onto face and neck area. Let dry for thirty minutes. Rinse with warm water.

Another interesting recipe comes to us from the South.

WHITE WINE CUCUMBER WRINKLE REMOVER

¼ cup	chopped cucumber
1	egg white
2 tablespoons	mayonnaise
2 ounces	fruit kernel oil
2 tablespoons	white wine
1	vitamin E capsule

1. In a blender combine the cucumber, egg white, mayonnaise, oil, and wine. Mix until well blended.
2. Pierce the vitamin E capsule, add contents to blender and mix thoroughly.
   • Massage into skin twice a day.

LOIRE ANTI-WRINKLER LOTION

Cucumbers contain a very effective anti-wrinkle enzyme. French women have relied on a cucumber anti-wrinkle lotion for generations to preserve their beautiful complexions.

1	cucumber
½ cup	rosé wine
1 tablespoon	anhydrous lanolin
2 ounces	comfrey root water
2 500-unit	vitamin E capsules

1. Slice the cucumber into the blender.
2. Add the rosé wine and liquefy.
3. Strain liquid through a clean cheesecloth into a glass bowl.
4. Melt the lanolin, then remove from heat and add the comfrey root water; beat until cool.
5. Add the cucumber-wine solution and continue beating until well mixed.
6. Puncture the vitamin E capsules and add.
   • Use daily before you go to bed.

PROTEIN WRINKLE REMOVER

Wrinkles and tiny facial lines disappear when bathed in a rich protein bath. The Protein Wrinkle Remover nourishes, stimulates, and tightens the skin. As the mask dries, the years seem to melt away.

2 teaspoons	soy protein powder
1 teaspoon	egg yolk
1 teaspoon	water
1 teaspoon	white wine

1. Combine all ingredients.
   - Spread a thin layer over the face and throat. Lie down and let dry for 30 minutes. Try not to talk or move your facial muscles during this time. Rinse with warm water, then cool. Pat dry. (If your skin feels slightly dry, massage in a small amount of nut oil.)

UNDER-EYE BAGS

The fragile under-eye tissue should be treated with special care. The area is especially susceptible to dry, tight skin due to the low oil content of the tissues. The skin should never be massaged or rubbed, but only lightly patted. Many people develop dark "bags" under their eyes despite good complexions. Our eyes mirror the health condition of our bodies, and fatigue quickly produces dark, ugly bags in the sensitive tissues beneath the eyes.

Another common complaint is swollen dark pockets that stretch the delicate under-eye tissue, Whatever the cause, most people want the complaint corrected as soon as possible. People with olive complexions often accept dark circles under their eyes, but they shouldn't. Dark circles are not natural and no one need suffer from embarrassing bags or circles anymore.

2	papaya tea bags
2 cups	boiling water
½ cup	dry white wine

1. Boil the water and wine together.
2. Let the tea bags steep until mixture cools to lukewarm.
   - Lie down, elevate your feet, and apply the tea bags to the area under your eyes for 15–20 minutes.

From Spain, famous for beautiful women, comes another interesting remedy for under-eye bags and circles. This remedy produces excellent results.

1	fresh fig
2 tablespoons	white wine
1 teaspoon	olive oil

1. Cut the fig in half.
2. Soak halves in wine for 30 minutes.
   - Apply the figs to the under-eye area for 10 minutes. Remove and gently pat in olive oil.

Here is a jet-set remedy for tightening sagging under-eye tissues. This simple, instant glamour secret can temporarily take off years.

| 1 | unbeaten egg white |
| 1 teaspoon | white wine |

The secret of success of this cure is to thin the unbeaten egg white down with the wine. Smooth on a thin layer of the mixture with your fingertips. Let dry, and then apply your make-up. Don't forget to follow the removal of your make-up with an olive oil pat, because the egg white and wine mixture can be very drying.

Why spend a fortune on chemically produced eye creams when this Swiss eye cream is super at only pennies a day?

SWISS EYE WRINKLE REDUCER

1 oz.	lanolin
1 oz.	white wine
½ oz.	almond oil
½ oz.	apricot kernel oil (found in most health food stores)
2500 units	Vitamin E

1. In a small pan melt the lanolin.
2. Add the wine, almond and apricot oils, and Vitamin E.
3. Pour while still warm into a small glass jar.
   - Each night gently pat into the delicate tissues around the eye to help reduce lines and wrinkles.

CROW'S FEET

Squinting, laughing, crying, frowning, all leave their imprint on the face, but emotion lines need not be permanent. "Laugh lines" begin appearing during the early twenties and slowly deepen into crow's feet during the following decade.

For instant improvement, try this ironing-out exercise and cream.

LINE BANISHER

Combine two ounces of nut oil (almond oil is excellent) and 1 tablespoon of red wine. Shake well before each application. Rub lightly into offending area. Take the palm of your hand and press firmly into the lined are for 1 minute, then relax the pressure. Repeat 3–4 times daily until lines begin to fade.

SWEDISH CURE

Very often crow's feet develop as the skin in the problem area begins to sag. To tighten the delicate skin in this area, follow this famous Swedish cure: Combine 1 teaspoon of honey, 1 teaspoon of unbeaten egg white, and ½ teaspoon of rosé wine. Beat together for 1–2 minutes. Pat on a thin layer around the eyes. Allow to dry for 5–10 minutes. Do not squint. Rinse with warm water. Pat, never rub, dry.

FRECKLES

By whatever name—freckles, sun kisses, or the Kiss of Apollo—these tiny brown blotches have caused many tears. Fortunately, freckles are more readily accepted in our informal society. But if your face is befreckled, you may feel differently and want to try fading your freckles. There are two basic types of freckles: the more permanent winter freckles and the summer freckles that intensify after exposure to the sun. To fade both freckle types, try the following four cures:

- To remove those ugly brown, café au lait spots from the skin, mix one-half teaspoon of onion juice with one teaspoon of white wine. Use as a wash.
- Mix ½ teaspoon onion juice with 1 teaspoon white wine. Use as a wash.
- Mix ¼ cup buttermilk with 2 tablespoons white wine. Spread on freckled area. Wait for 10 minutes and rinse with warm water. Results become visible only after a month's daily use. Don't be discouraged; buttermilk is an excellent skin bleach.
- Every night, rub white wine on the freckles. Do not rinse until morning. If dryness develops, rub on a thin layer of nut oil.

FACIAL SKIN HEMORRHAGES

Those tiny red lines that mar your complexion are a definite problem. The spidery lines are caused by ruptured delicate blood vessel walls. Victorian beauties jealously guarded the following secret cure for this cosmetic misery.

STRAWBERRY REFRESHER

Strawberries are rich in bioflavinoids that are successfully used to treat skin hemorrhages. Fresh, ripe strawberries are essential to this remedy.

½ pound	fresh, ripe strawberries
½ teaspoon	corn starch
1 teaspoon	rosé wine

1. Mash the strawberries in a glass bowl.
2. Combine the wine and corn starch until a paste is formed. Add to berries.
3. Stir the strawberry and paste mixture over low heat for five minutes. Cool.
4. Pout into a covered jar and store in refrigerator.
   • Massage a small amount of the mixture into the skin every evening. Rinse in the morning with warm water. *Caution:* Strawberries may stain linen, so consider using an old pillowcase. As only fresh strawberries are effective in the mixture, during strawberry season large quantities of it may be prepared and frozen.

BATH BEAUTIFIERS

For centuries, Swiss women have believed in the power of oats, not only as a rewarding beauty food rich in the minerals magnesium, potassium, and phosphorus plus vitamins B and E, but as a healthy beauty bath that lets the body slowly soak up these nutrients. Oatmeal baths replenish important skin oils and provide a protective screen that not only softens but gently bleaches the skin to a milky white sheen.

OATMEAL BEAUTY BATH

1 cup	natural oatmeal
1 cup	dry white wine
3 cups	water

1. In a blender grind the oatmeal to a fine powder.
2. Add wine to blender and let the mixture marinate for 30 minutes.
3. Warm the water and add to the wine and oatmeal mixture and blend on low speed for 3 minutes.
4. Strain the fluid through a fine sieve or gauze into a jar.
5. Fill a small porous bag or straining gauze with the remaining oats.

6. Fill the bathtub halfway with hot, steamy water and add the strained oatmeal and wine liquid.
7. Use the small bag of oats in the water as a washcloth.
- Bathe daily, using the mixture rather than commercially prepared soap for 1 month. A new soft look to your skin should be noticeable within the first week.

For the last several years everyone has sung the praises of bran, but Colonial women knew that bran was an excellent remedy for dry skin. Fill a small muslin bag with bran and soak it for several minutes in white wine. Place in hot bathwater and use as a washcloth all over your body for a delightful tingly sensation.

ECZEMA

Eczema is one of the most common and frustrating skin conditions. The most important point to remember about eczema is that it is the result of skin that is easily damaged, especially by chemicals, soap, and other caustic drying agents.

BATH OIL

A Danish dermatologist highly recommends this bath oil to soothe delicate skin tissues.

1 oz.	crushed comfrey root*
1 oz.	echinacea or goldenseal*
1 oz.	white willow bark*
½ cup	dry white wine
1 qt.	vegetable oil
1	fresh onion, chopped
1 cup	wheat germ oil

Ingredients found at the health food store

1. Place the herbs in a large metal pan and add the wine.
2. Simmer for 1 hour.
3. Add vegetable oil and onion, bring to a boil and simmer until wine evaporates (approximately 20 minutes).
4. Cool.

5. Strain through a cheesecloth until the oil is clear and the sediment is at the bottom.

6. Decant the oil infusion and add the wheat germ oil.

- Rub the finished moisturizing oil on your skin daily, or use as a soothing bath oil.

DANISH ITCH LOTION

3 tablespoons	white wine
1 teaspoon	fresh horseradish
1 cup	yogurt

1. Grate horseradish into wine.

2. Let stand for 15 minutes.

3. Combine with yogurt.

4. Refrigerate the mixture for 2 days and then strain out the grated horseradish.

- Dab on the mixture until relief is felt. Rinse with cold water. Pat dry.

TANNING

The sun, while essential to life and health, is the skin's worst enemy. Moderate amounts are acceptable, but overindulgence is definitely a danger to your health. Overexposure will cause dry, leathery skin that can age you years in several months.

But with the first warm days of summer, people insist on sunbathing. The dry-cooked, weathered cowboy look seems to be a status symbol during the warm weather but leaves the complexion with as much life as a tanned animal hide. If you ever traveled on the Riviera, you must have noticed that Frenchwomen, although they enjoy the sun, still manage to have soft, supple skin.

The following two skin creams will allow you to acquire a soft suntan while screening out the majority of the harmful ultraviolet rays. Both creams should give you more protection than many of the chemically produced commercial products. Enjoy the sun, but treat it with respect! As the Noel Coward song says, "Mad dogs and Englishmen go out in the mid-day sun."

ST. TROPEZ SUNTANNING CREAM

1 tablespoon	red wine
½ cup	sesame seed oil
1	egg yolk
1 teaspoon	mint juice (mint leaf extract)

1. In a blender, combine all ingredients until thick.
2. Store in an opaque jar.
3. Keep refrigerated when not in use.

RIVIERA SUN CREAM

3 tablespoons	white wine
4 ozs.	plain natural yogurt
1 tablespoon	potato flour
2 tablespoons	avocado oil
2 tablespoons	sunflower seed oil
2 tablespoons	safflower oil
6 tablespoons	water dispersible lecithin
2 tablespoons	sesame oil

1. Combine all ingredients in a blender.
2. Mix until smooth.
3. Keep refrigerated when not in use.

CREAMY TAHITIAN TAN

1 oz.	cocoa butter
1 oz.	sesame oil
2 ozs.	coconut oil
1 teaspoon	red wine

1. Combine all ingredients.
2. Mix thoroughly.

MAYONNAISE TANNING CREAM

Take ½ cup mayonnaise, preferably fresh or purchased at a health food store, and add 2 tablespoons white wine. The wine hastens the tan and affords extra protection from the sun.

SUNBURN

If you are suffering from an uncomfortable sunburn, you need effective relief now. The most effective sunburn healer is the Aloe Cooler. Scoop out the center gel-like substance from the aloe leaf. Mix until spreadable with one or two drops of red wine. Spread over the sunburn.

Other super sunburn coolers include:

- Cucumber slices soaked in white wine
- Apple cider vinegar and white wine compresses
- Natural yogurt diluted with white wine
- Witch hazel diluted with white wine

BARLEY PASTE

3 ounces	unpearled barley
1 tablespoon	red wine
1 ounce	raw honey
1	unbeaten egg white

1. In the blender grind the barley into a powder.
2. Add the wine and let soak for 2 minutes.
3. Mix in the honey and egg white until the ingredients are the consistency of a smooth paste.
- Rub gently onto sunburned areas and leave overnight.

HAND CARE

Any season or occupation can be hard on your hands. Housework can produce rough raw hands that can be extremely painful. Daily skin care is extremely important to protect your hands. An evening application of the following moisturizing cream will restore or protect overused or abused hands: In a double boiler melt a one-ounce cake of white beeswax. Blend in two ounces of sweet almond oil and one ounce of dry white wine. Remove from heat and pour immediately into a covered jar. Apply nightly or before going out in cold weather.

118

Equal amounts of fresh tomato juice and red wine make an excellent hand massage. It is especially good for the cuticles.

Supple smooth hands are not an unattainable dream. Try combining one ounce of honey with one egg white and one teaspoon of white wine with ground barley. Rub the mixture into hands daily.

Frenchwomen are famous for long, luscious nails. To strengthen your own nails, fill a small bottle with castor oil and add four drops of white iodine and four drops of white wine. Shake well before each application. Paint your nails twice daily with the mixture.

HEALTHY SHINING HAIR

Hair has been described as the crowning glory of beauty. Millions of dollars are spent yearly trying to thicken, straighten, curl, and color our tresses. Healthy hair is a precious beauty asset, and can be achieved simply and inexpensively by daily loving care with natural herbs and wine.

SHAMPOOS

You can hardly turn on the TV or flip a page in a magazine without being faced with an advertisement about shampoos. The popular herbal shampoos have captured the market lead, but how much does the consumer actually know about the materials used to synthesize the herbal ingredients? Are the so-called "organic" or "natural" shampoos commercially formulated with artificial and potentially dangerous chemicals? Is there any need to be sucked in by exaggerated advertising promises? Or can the consumer substitute natural substances with outstanding results?

BRANDY SHAMPOO FOR NORMAL HAIR

From France, where women of fashion are famous for knowledgeable hair care, comes the brandy/egg shampoo cure. This shampoo is famous for giving dull, limp locks life and body.

The basic ingredients are ¼ cup brandy and 1 egg yolk.

Beat together for several minutes and apply to dry hair that has been well brushed. Massage mixture into scalp and hair for seven minutes. Rinse with warm water and towel dry.

EGG WASH

France also gives us the egg/wine wash for split, lifeless, flyaway locks. The luxurious treatment will rival any $50 salon hot oil treatment for just pennies. The egg yolks nourish the roots while the wine helps assimilate the protein to the hair strands. The egg yolk/wine combination is truly the dynamic duo of hair care.

1 teaspoon	dry white wine
1 cup	warm water
2	egg yolks

1. Combine the wine and warm water.
2. Mix in the egg yolks.
   - Massage mixture into hair and scalp. Cover hair with a plastic bag and secure ends. (This will quicken protein assimiliation to the hair shafts.) Leave the bag in place for 10 minutes. Pour ¼ cup of warm water over head and massage into lather. Rinse with warm water. The final touch: Pour 1 tablespoon dry white wine into a quart of warm water and rinse hair throughly. Towel dry.

MINT PICK-ME-UP SHAMPOO

This is the perfect cure for dull, lifeless, wind- and sun-damaged hair. Eggs are an important source of protein for the body and are instrumental in repairing lifeless, damaged hair. Combined with mint, they cleanse, rejuvenate, and strengthen the hair shafts. The Mint-Pick-Me-Up Shampoo cure should be followed two or three times weekly for a month.

1 handful	fresh mint leaves
2 tablespoons	white wine
1 cup	boiling water
2	egg yolks

1. Crush the mint leaves in a bowl.
2. Add the wine.
3. Add the boiling water and let steep for 15 minutes.
4. Strain out the mint leaves and reserve the mint/wine liquid.
5. Beat the egg yolks until frothy and add to the liquid.
6. Mix together well.
   • Massage into scalp for 5–10 minutes. Rinse with warm water.

FOR OILY HAIR ONLY

This treatment should cut down the need for excessive shampoos. Shampoo twice with an herbal shampoo, paying close attention to massaging the scalp. For the final rinse, make up a solution of 1 quart warm water to which has been added 2 tablespoons white wine. Towel dry.

BASIC BEAUTY SHAMPOO

The majority of Americans overshampoo, causing dull, lifeless, hair. To repair the hair try the following special care shampoo and rinse.

1. Wet the hair with very warm water. This opens the pores.
2. Slowly pour a small amount of your regular shampoo over your scalp.
3. Gently but firmly massage your scalp with your finger pads, not your fingernails, for 5 minutes.
4. Rinse with warm water.
5. Apply more shampoo and lather hair.
6. Rinse thoroughly.
7. Apply wine rinse or herbal wine rinse.

WINE RINSE

Helps stimulate the scalp, increases the flow of natural oils that help repair dry, split ends.

Take 1 tablespoon white wine and mix with 2 cups of warm water.

If you would prefer an herbal rinse, try one of the following:

1. Combine herbs (see below)—approximately 1–4 table-spoons. Place in covered non-metal pot and add 1 cup of cold water.
2. Add 2 tablespoons wine, bring contents to boil, reduce heat and simmer for 5 minutes.
3. Strain out herbs and add 1 cup cold water to remaining liquid infusion. The reserved herbs make excellent plant food.
4. Pour the infusion over the head and massage gently into scalp. Hair may be rinsed with cool water, but it is not necessary.

Dry hair: Combine equal amounts of elder flower, acacia (one of the most fragrant flowers used in making perfume), comfrey root, clover, and orange blossoms with 2 tablespoons red wine.

To brighten dark hair: Combine equal amounts of chamomile, marigold flowers, henna, and rosemary with 2 tablespoons of white wine.

Light hair: Combine equal amounts of marigold flowers, chamomile, orange peel, and yellow mullein flowers with 2 tablespoons of rosé wine, *or* combine equal amounts of marigold, acacia flowers, and chamomile with 2 tablespoons of white wine.

Dandruff rinse: Any of the following herbal rinses combined with 2 tablespoons of red wine will considerably improve dandruff conditions: artichoke leaves, birch bark, nettle, or white willow bark.

Oily hair: Combine equal amounts of lemon peel, willow bark, lemon grass, and quassia chips with 3 tablespoons white wine.

Dry, itchy scalp: Make a rinse from birch bark and witch hazel with 2 tablespoons of red wine.

During the past decade, an increasing number of people have been suffering from thinning hair. Many dermatologists feel that chemically concocted shampoos and rinses are at fault. If you have noticed an increase in falling hair, try the following rinse:

3 ozs.	rosemary leaves
1 teaspoon	baking soda
½ teaspoon	camphor
1 teaspoon	red wine
1 quart	spring water
4 ozs.	rum

1. In a saucepan combine the first four ingredients with the water and bring to a boil.
2. Remove from heat.
3. Strain and add the rum.
   • Massage the infusion into the roots daily.

BASIC WINE RINSE

The basic wine rinse is excellent for softening and conditioning the hair while neutralizing the alkalinity of soap. Any herbs can be used in the basic wine rinse by following the basic seven steps.

1. Combine the desired herbs.
2. Bring 1 cup of dry white wine to a boil in a metal saucepan and pour over approximately 1 ounce of the herb mixture.
3. Pour mixture into a covered glass jar and store in a cool, dark place for at least 1 week. Shake daily.
4 .Strain out the herbs and reserve the herbal wine mixture.
5. After shampooing, mix 1 tablespoon of the wine mixture with 1 cup warm water.
6. Massage into scalp.
7. Rinse with cool water.

FOR BLONDES ONLY

To lighten blond hair, try these secrets from Scandinavia.
   Beat two egg whites until very stiff. After having brushed your hair for ten minutes, rub into the scalp three tablespoons white wine. This will stimulate the pores. Then, with

light circular strokes, massage in the beaten egg whites. Dry your hair in the sun for twenty minutes, or, in winter, for ten or fifteen minutes under a sun lamp. Brush to shining luster.

Another Nordic lightening secret is to wash the hair every other week in a half-and-half mixture of ale and white wine.

DAMAGED, OVER DYED HAIR

Dyeing, bleaching, and stripping can leave your hair a disaster. Even expensive salon treatments often cannot counteract the years of abuse.

From Spain comes an interesting remedy that should generate immediate results:

1. Warm approximately ¼ cup olive oil and massage into both hair and scalp for 5 minutes. Comb through hair to insure entire coating of strands. Cover hair with a plastic bag for 1 hour to contain scalp heat and promote proper saturation. Shampoo oil away with an herbal shampoo. More than one application may be necessary. Rinse twice with a mixture of 3 tablespoons of red wine and 1 quart warm water. Towel dry; do not blow-dry.
2. Prepare the second-step shampoo by beating 2 eggs with 2 tablespoons of red wine. Massage into the hair and leave on for 20 minutes before rinsing with clear warm water. Towel dry.
3. Combine ½ cup mayonnaise, 1 egg, and 1 tablespoon of red wine. Massage the mixture into the hair and let stand for 1 hour. Shampoo with an herbal shampoo and rinse with a mixture of 2 cups warm water and 2 tablespoons of red wine.

From Italy comes another interesting dry hair comditioning treatment.

CONDITIONER

Slice a ripe avocado into the blender. Add 3 tablespoons of red wine, and blend until the mixture has the consistency of a thick paste. Massage the mixture into hair and scalp for 10 minutes. Cover the hair with a plastic bag for 1 hour. Rinse with a mixture of 1 quart of warm water and 3 tablespoons of red wine. Towel dry.

PROTEIN SHAMPOO

A rich protein shampoo is essential to help dry hair. Beat 2 egg yolks and 2 teaspoons of red wine in ¼ cup warm water. Massage mixture into scalp. Rinse with warm water.

BALDNESS

The mere mention of the word makes strong men quake with fear. Millions are spent annually by men who refuse to submit to a receding hairline or balding head. Is there hope? Can a simple compound made at home prevent baldness and stimulate hair growth? You be the judge.

From southern Europe, where men are famous for thick, luscious hair, come the following growth stimulators:

CURE I:

1 cup	olive oil
1 teaspoon	dried marjoram
1 teaspoon	rosemary oil
1 teaspoon	red wine

Combine all the ingredients and rub into the roots daily.

CURE II:

1 oz.	olive oil
1 oz.	rosemary oil
½ oz.	nutmeg oil (approximately 8–10 drops)
½ oz.	red wine

Combine all the ingredients and massage the mixture into the scalp every night. Brush the hair vigorously twice daily with a small amount of oil of rosemary.

CURE III:

In a food processor, powder peach kernels (available at your health food store). Store the powder in a covered jar. Take 2 ounces of the powdered peach kernels and add 8 ounces of boiling red wine. Store in a dark place for two weeks. Then massage the infusion into the scalp daily.

HOW TO THICKEN YOUR HAIR

Thin, lifeless hair is a number one beauty problem, not only for women but for men. If you want added fullness, try this old-time French treatment, praised for generations for its effectiveness.

FRENCH HAIR TREATMENT

4 tablespoons	rosemary
½ pound	raw honey
1 quart	white wine
¼ pint	sweet almond oil

1. Mix the rosemary, honey, and wine together.
2. Boil for 5 minutes, reduce heat, and add almond oil.
3. Pour into a covered glass jar.
   • Daily massage mixture into the roots.

SAGE/WINE HAIR TONIC I

A simple infusion of sage combined with equal parts of rosemary and red wine is said to stimulate the growth of hair. Keep in the refrigerator and use twice daily.

SAGE/WINE HAIR TONIC II

In France, to condition and darken gray hair, many men use a sage-wine tonic.

2 heaping teaspoons sage
2 heaping teaspoons tea, any
  type
½ cup red wine
1 cup boiling water
1 tablespoon brandy

1. In a pint container, combine sage and tea.
2. Add boiling water and wine.
3. Cover and place in slow oven for two hours. (The solution should darken.)
4. Remove and strain.
5. Add brandy.
   • Rub the lotion into hair roots every night.

LUSCIOUS LASHES

To stimulate the growth of long, luscious eyelashes, apply this long-known folk remedy.

1 cup   olive oil
1 tablespoon   red wine

1. Combine oil and wine.
2. Store in covered jar and shake before each application.
   • With a cotton swab, rub the eyelashes with the mixture. Be sure to put it only on your eyelashes and not the eyelids.

HERBAL MASSAGE

I was first introduced to the benefits of the hot herbal massage in Sweden by a woman who was in her late sixties, looked thirty, and had the energy of a teenager. She reluctantly told me the secret of preparing the oil at home, and although initially it may seem complicated, the results are well worth the effort.

The following formulas are to help sagging breasts, remove cellulite, and trim limbs, and are so successful that you will become an instant hot herbal oil convert.

THE BASIC METHOD

1. Select a non-metal 3-quart pot and add approximately 4 ounces of the selected herbs.
2. Add ½ cup dry white wine to the herbs and let stand for 2 to 3 hours. The wine you select should have a high alcohol content, at least 10 percent, as it is the alcohol that extracts the actual substance from the herbs.
3. Add 2 quarts of vegetable oil to the mixture.
4. Cover the pan and simmer until all the wine has cooked off. As the wine evaporates you will begin to smell the aroma of the herbs.
5. Let the oil cool and then strain through cheesecloth into a covered container. Store in a dark place for 7 days. Do not disturb during this period as the oil is settling.
6. Decant the remaining clear oil and discard the residue. One ounce of your favorite essential oil may be added to the massage oil at this time.

HOT HERBAL MASSAGE OIL FOR SAGGING BREASTS

1 oz.	woodruff
1 oz.	lady's mantle
1 oz.	quince seed
1 oz.	comfrey leaf

1. Follow Basic Method using above herbs.
2. Scent with pure vanilla oil—it smells best and also tastes good. This oil is considered extremely erotic and sensual.
   • Massage nightly into breasts. Starting at the outside using your thumbs, work in a circular movement under and around the breast up to the nipples.

A simplified version of the hot herbal massage comes from southern Italy, where women preserve their breasts with time-honored restorers: germ oil, red wine, and vanilla.

Heat a mixture of equal amounts of the wine and germ oil until warm, scent with vanilla, and massage as above.

CELLULITE

Several years ago, beauty experts made us aware of cellulite, and since that time women around the world have been trying to rid themselves of ugly pockets of fat.

Massage is extremely important in breaking down the gel-like fat deposits. The Zürich doctor I talked to has his patients run very hot water directly from the tap over the affected knee, hip, or thigh areas before massage. The force of the water, he felt, played an important part in the fat breakdown.

One French doctor I met prescribed special herbal-wine diuretic teas to help relieve cellulite by the elimination of waste products from the tissues. Whatever method you select, from baths to hot massages, to cure your cellulite problem, you should notice a significant improvement and begin to feel better almost immediately.

HOT OIL HERBAL MASSAGE METHOD

Follow the basic hot oil steps on page 150.

Massage 1: Combine equal amounts of chamomile, marigold, witch hazel leaves, and scent with ¼ oz. lemon essential oil.
Massage 2: Combine one ounce each of pennyroyal, orange leaves, linden, and scent with ¼ ounce of mint oil.
Massage 3: Combine one ounce each of sage and jaborandi, two ounces of strawberry leaves, and scent with ¼ ounce sage oil.

• Massage with a kneading action daily into cellulite-affected areas.

FRENCH CELLULITE MASSAGE OIL

1 oz.	lemon oil
½ oz.	lime oil
3 ozs.	almond oil
3 ozs.	vodka
3 ozs.	red wine

1. Mix together the oils.
2. Add the vodka and red wine.

- Massage with strong strokes to remove cellulite. In France, this massage oil is used exclusively in elegant body salons. Many Paris showgirls rely on this massage treatment to keep their figures sensational.

French models exclusively use a lemon grass and wine massage to improve circulation and reduce fluid buildup which leads to a cellulite problem. Combine 1 ounce of essential oil of lemon grass and 3 ounces of vodka and 1 ounce of white wine. Massage twice daily, in the morning and the evening.

MIRACLE FAT REMOVAL BATH

Fill a bathtub with very hot water and pour in 1 pound of Epsom salts and 2 cups of white wine. Make a salt scrub by pouring some salt into a muslin cloth and tying the ends. With strong strokes, rub down your entire body. Now soak in the tub for 30 minutes.

HERBAL FAT SOAK

Another intriguing Scandinavian remedy is the herbal fat soak. In this method, a hot herbal compress is applied directly to the fatty areas and then followed by a herbal bath.

1 oz.	thyme
1 oz.	seaweed
1 oz.	jaborandi
2 cups	water
2 cups	white wine

1. Simmer ingredients for 15 minutes in a non-metal pan.
2. Strain herbs.
   - Apply herbs to fatty areas while still warm. Pour the remaining liquid into a hot bath and soak for 30 minutes.

Special note: Jaborandi leaves are poisonous if taken internally. Commercially, jaborandi is used in shampoos, herbal hair rinses, but its most important application is in body lotions to help stimulate the pores. When used in a herbal wine bath, jaborandi acts as a powerful diuretic that rids the body of excess water.

FLABBY SKIN CARE

Dieting and exercise alone cannot tighten flabby flesh and return the skin to its former tone. Special care should be given to trouble spots which need extra attention. One of the most common after-diet complaints is flabby upper arms and sagging fannies. To firm these weakened areas, try daily massage with the following:

FANTASTIC FIRMING LOTION

1	cucumber
3 teaspoons	tincture of benzoin
¼ cup	white wine
¼ cup	warm water

1. Liquefy cucumber (including skin unless heavily waxed) in a blender.
2. Strain off 5 tablespoons juice.
3. In a glass jar, combine juice with remaining ingredients.
4. Refrigerate.
   • Massage into troubled areas several times daily.

A famous French actress, who wishes to remain anonymous, mixes together equal amounts of dried skim milk, egg whites, and white wine to form a paste that tightens the skin of the neck.

PART THREE

BUYING WINES FOR YOUR HEALTH

CHAPTER TEN

BUYING WINES FOR YOUR HEALTH

Wine stores, with their floor-to-ceiling displays of imported bottles, can be intimidating to all except the wine snob. Fortunately, with a little study and sampling, anyone can become a fairly competent wine connoisseur. You say you can't afford it? Nonsense! I know the wine experts enjoy singing the praises of Château Latour '61 or Steinberger Riesling Trockenbeerenauslese '59, granted they were superb vintages for a privileged few, but the healing properties of these wines are no better than the hundreds of more affordable brands.

More than 90 percent of all wine consumed in the U.S. costs only about $4.00 a bottle. Of course, if paying $20 and up makes you feel better, by all means, do so, but don't expect to feel five times as good. California has increased planting, resulting in a vast number of high-quality new labels. Americans are demanding consumers; they know quality and want to drink the wine, not pay for the label. Today's economy has produced more discriminating buyers who know the taste, smell, and look of a good wine, and want one that fits their budgetary limits. More and more American and imported wines are meeting these criteria.

In a recent blind tasting, the experts tasted several American and French white wines. The expensive French wine placed last. The winner was an American wine that cost only $1.25 for a 25.6-ounce bottle. This is not a condemnation of French wines, of which I happen to be very fond, but an example of how the experts—the wine snobs with their trained palates—can often be wrong.

Shopping around is the key to success in finding wine bargains. As with generic drugs, liquor stores can vary as much as 30 percent on the price of the same wine. Recently, I found a German Kabinett selling for $3.50 in one store and $2.25 in another! I keep a small notebook to record, rate, and list new wines. Keeping a record is essential to sorting out and understanding the myriad of wines on today's market.

We are extremely fortunate in the United States to have such a wide variety of wine from around the world from which to choose. On a recent trip to a local liquor store, I found wines from France, Germany, Spain, Italy, Portugal, Israel, Australia, Yugoslavia, Canada, Czechoslovakia, Argentina, Denmark, South Africa, Bulgaria, Hungary, Greece, Mexico, Morocco, and the United States!

In California alone there are more than eight thousand different wines on the market. No single retailer could ever stock such a bewildering variety, but most wine store operators are knowledgeable and willing to help advise you on your purchases. But don't stop here. Wine store safaris are fun, profitable, and extremely valuable in gaining knowledge.

You are the final judge! In the last analysis, you have to decide what wine is best to drink for your health.

Let's begin by evaluating some reasonably priced wines available on the American market in comparison with their European counterparts.

HOW TO APPRECIATE A GOOD WINE

Wine relates to the five senses!

Smell it. The bouquet should be pleasing to the nose.
See it. The color, the body, should be appealing to the eye.
Hear it. To toast a friend, to clink your glass, is pleasing to the ear. The winegrowers of Alsace say, "You feel for the bottle, and when you find a good one, you can hear the angels sing."
Feel it. A good wine delights the senses; its texture is velvet in the mouth.
Taste it. The final glory is the taste on the tongue.

WHITE WINES

Grape Variety	Californian	European	Notes
Chardonnay	Called Pinot Chardonnay or Chardonnay.	Found in parts of Italy and in France in Burgundy, Chablis, and Champagne.	High-quality, low-yield production. Top American wines can favorably compare with the best French Burgundies.
Chenin Blanc	Best growths found in Monterey, Napa, San Benito, Santa Clara, and Sonoma counties.	Native to the Loire Valley.	Used to produce many California Champagne blends.
Colombard	Grown in upper central valley and north coast areas.	Used in producing the great brandy of France.	The California grape is lower in acid than its French counterpart, producing light dry wine, although it is sometimes on the sweet side.
Folle Blanche	Grown in the central valley and north coast areas.	Produces a light white wine in many of the French provinces.	In California this grape makes a wonderfully refreshing wine with a slight tart taste.

WHITE WINES *(Continued)*

Grape Variety	Californian	European	Notes
Gewürztraminer	Grows best in north coast area.	Grown in northern Italy, Alsace, and Germany.	Both European and American varieties offer the same great-tasting wines.
Johannisberg Riesling	Grows best in a cave climate, especially in the north counties.	Grown in Austria, Luxembourg, northern Italy and Germany, primarily in the Mosel and Rhine valleys.	The word "Johannisberg" only appears on true Riesling grapes in California This is a milder taste than its cousins.
Sauvignon Blanc	Grown in upper central valley and north coast areas.	Grown in France in Graves, Sauternes, and Loire Valley.	Sold in California as Blanc-Fumé or California Dry Sauterne. The wine is similar to French Graves.
Barbera	Grown in Napa, Sonoma and warmer regions of the central valley.	Native to northern Italy.	Superior quality produced in Napa and Sonoma counties, often better than Italian vari-

RED WINES

Grape Variety	Californian	European	Notes
			ety. Central valley growth has not proven itself yet.
Cabernet Sauvignon	Found along the north coast.	Prominent in Bordeaux vineyards.	Although not up to the best French red Bordeaux, definitely the best California red wine.
Gamay	Grows best in the warmer central valley and north coast, but called Napa Gamay.	Grown in many European vineyards. Best found in Beaujolais.	High-volume grape producing a light middle-of-the-road wine. Pleasing, not outstanding. Do not confuse this grape with Gamay Beaujolais.
Gamay Beaujolais	Found planted from northern Mendocino to southern Monterey counties	Not grown in Europe.	Strain of the Pinot Noir grape.

RED WINES *(Continued)*

Grape Variety	Californian	European	Notes
Grenache	Responsible for the best California port production. Also used in central valley jug wine and north coast rosés.	Tavel rosé grape, planted in parts of the Châteauneuf-du-Pape, major parts of the Côtes du Rhône, and the Rioja of Spain.	California's rosé and red jug wines owe their good quality to the Grenache grape.
Pinot Noir	Found in the Mendocino, Napa and Sonoma counties in limited quantity due to high production cost and low yield.	All Burgundy wines of France contain 100% of this noble grape.	Not as good as California Cabernet Sauvignon.
Zinfandel	Unique to California. Best growths found in north coast counties.	Unknown.	America's best jug wines are based on this grape.

CHAPTER ELEVEN

EUROPEAN WINES

WINES OF FRANCE

France can still claim to be the greatest wine-producing country in the world, though Italy has more acres planted in vineyards and weather conditions in some years permit Italy to produce more wines.

With good weather France can produce up to 1,600,000,000 gallons of wine each year. This wine is divided into three classes: A.C., *Appellations contrôlées;* V.D.Q.S., *Vins délimités de qualité supérieure;* and V.C.C., *Vins de consommation courante.*

A.C. wines are fine wines, which bear a regional name and have been made according to rigid rules to insure proper alcoholic content. V.D.Q.S. wines are regional wines of fairly good quality, and are beginning to deserve more of the connoisseur's atention. V.C.C. are ordinary regional wines that up until several years ago were not exported in quantity. Today V.C.C. wines are enjoying a favorable market share in competition with many of the American jug wines.

BORDEAUX—BORDEAUX SUPÉRIEUR

Fourteen Bordeaux appellations are sold not under their own appellations, but as Bordeaux or Bordeaux Supérieur, including such well-known names as Premières Côtes de Bordeaux,

Côtes de Blaye, and Côte de Castillon. The simple Bordeaux wines are pleasant, light, basic red wines, while wines grown in the Médoc, Saint-Émilion, and Graves districts are usually fuller and have more style and elegance.

The vineyards of the Bordeaux region are perhaps the oldest of France, dating back to Imperial Rome. For the next twenty centuries, the Bordeaux region was a major wine-producing area, with over 300,000 acres of vineyards. The soil of the various areas is rich in limestone, silica, iron, and potassium. It is these individual elements that are so very important in the medicinal effects of Bordeaux wines.

Saint-Émilion wines are considered especially effective in treating menopause, hemorrhage, fatigue, and arthritis. Wines from the Médoc are most effective against tonsillitis and other throat infections, salmonella, nephritis, tuberculosis, osteoporosis, allergies, diarrhea, diabetes, depression, and bronchitis. Graves wines are especially good for appetite control and anemia.

RECOMMENDED WINES:

Red	White
La Cour Pavillon	Lichine Graves
Lichine Médoc	Mouton-Cadet
Sichel My Cousin's Claret	Pontet-Latour
Ginestet Haut-Médoc	
B & G Prince Noir	
Pontet-Latour	
Mouton-Cadet	

For a greater variety, the consumer may want to sample wines imported from the following list of petits châteaux, which are not smaller vineyards, but lesser growths. Petits châteaux wines, unlike the great slow-maturing Bordeaux growths, can be bought young, drunk young, and provide the best wine value today.

- Blaye, Côtes de Blaye and Premières Côtes de Blaye. A fruity delicate wine meant to be drunk young. Try the Château Barbé red.
- Bourg, Bourgeais, and Côtes de Bourg. The red wines are hearty, fruity, full-bodied; the whites are slightly

sweet and often used in blending. Try wines from Châteaux Barbé and du Bousquet.

- Côtes Canon-Fronsac, Côtes de Fronsac. Excellent value, high-quality, long-lived red wines which store well for up to ten years. Try wines from Château Rouct or Château Canon.
- Entre-Deux-Mers. The white wines of this region are dry, fresh, and an exceptionally good value. The reds are sold as either Bordeaux or Bordeaux Supérieur.
- Graves, Graves de Vayres. Two-thirds of the wine produced in the area is white, dry with a slight sulphurous taste. Although not as popular as other white French wines, the quality is high and the price is less expensive. The reds of the area have a definite taste with good body. Try wines from Château Haut-Brion.
- Haut-Médoc, Médoc. Although both white and red wines are produced, due to strict quality control only the reds can display an A.C. The wines of the area are impressive, showing great strength and character. Try wines from several of the famous communes, Saint-Estéphe, Saint-Julien, Margaux, Pauillac.
- Listrac. The red wines of the area are slightly astringent when young, but age beautifully. Try wines from Château Fourcas-Hostein.
- Margaux. The wines of the area are smooth, silky, and well-bred. Although Château Margaux, a famous first great growth, is the reputed king, there are many wonderful petits châteaux from the area.
- Moulis. This small commune produces tannic red wines that age well in the bottle, but are wonderfully fruity and delicious when drunk young. Try wines from the Château Chasse-Spleen.
- Pauillac. This small commune produces reds that are dry, earthy, full-bodied. Many good petits châteaux are produced in the area.
- Pomerol, Lalande de Pomerol, Néac. The wines of this area are low in tannin and good when drunk young. The taste is soft and rich. Although the "classified growths" of this area are very expensive, there are extremely good bargains available from top-quality petits châteaux.
- Premières Côtes de Bordeaux. Although both red and white wines are produced, the whites account for the greater volume and are of a higher quality. The taste

ranges from semi-dry to sweet with many whites being favorably compared to Sauternes.
- Saint-Émilion. Here we find fruitier wines that mature faster and are pleasant when drunk young.

BURGUNDY

Although the Burgundy vineyards only produce about two percent of the total French wine volume, the proud Burgundians are secure in the knowledge that their wines are some of the finest in the world.

The two major grapes of the region are the Chardonnay and Pinot Noir. The Gamay grape is grown almost exclusively in the Beaujolais region.

Even more than other French wines, Burgundies are individuals. Their distinctive flavors vary from vineyard to vineyard. The great reds have attained an exquisite balance of flavor, fullness, bouquet, warmth, and fruitiness; the whites are wonderfully dry, fresh-tasting, full and well-balanced. Burgundies have been appreciated by gourmets for years.

Burgundy has five major wine-growing districts: Chablis, Côte de Nuits, Côte de Beaune, Chalonnais, and Mâconnais, and Beaujolais. The soil from the various districts varies in mineral composition, but the most important Beaujolais, Chablis, and Mâcon districts are noted for high soil deposits of silicon dioxide. The Côtes de Nuit, Côtes de Dijon, and Côte de Beaune grapes flourish in a limestone soil that is rich in iron.

Beaujolais wines are effective in treating bronchitis, tonsillitis, and diarrhea. Wines from the Côte de Beaune are recommended for fatigue, weight control, cardiac insufficiency, and anemia. The listings give the names of the communes and the vineyards within each district.

RECOMMENDED WINES:

CÔTE DE BEAUNE

Red

Aloxe-Corton
  ●Corton

White

Aloxe-Corton
  ●Corton-Charlemagne

●Corton-Grancey
●Clos du Roi
Auxey-Duresses

Auxey-Duresses
Beaune
  ●Le Clos-des-Mouches
Blanc

Red

Beaune
  ●Le Clos-des-Mouches
  ●Aux Cras
  ●Les Fèves
  ●Les Grèves
Pernand-Vergelesses
Pommard
Volnay
  ●En Caillerets
  ●Le Clos-des-Chênes
  ●Les Clos-des-Ducs

White

Chassagne-Montrachet
  ●La Boudriotte
  ●En Cailleret
  ●Criots-Bâtard-Montra-
  chet
  ●Montrachet
  ●Grandes-Ruchottes
  ●Monthélie
Puligny-Montrachet
  ●Le Cailleret
  ●Les Combettes
  ●Les Pucelles

CÔTE DE NUITS

Red

Chambolle-Musigny
  ●Les Amoureuses
  ●Les Charmes
Côte de Nuits Villages
Fixin
  ●Clos de la Perrière
  ●Clos Napoléon
Gevrey-Chambertin
  ●Aux Combottes
  ●Le Clos Saint-Jacques
  ●Griotte-Chambertin
  ●Les Véroilles
Morey-Saint Denis
  ●Clos-des-Lambrays
  ●Clos de la Roche
  ●Clos de Tart
Nuits-Saint-Georges
  ●Les Saint-Georges

White

Vosne-Romanée
  ●Les Malconsorts
  ●Les Suchots

- Les Porets
- Les Pruliers
- Les Vaucrains

BEAUJOLAIS

Red

Beaujolais
Beaujolais-Villages
Côte de Brouilly
Chénas
Chiroubles
Juliénas
Morgon
Saint-Amour

MÂCON

White

Mâcon Blanc
Pouilly-Vinzelles
Saint-Véran
Pouilly-Fuissé
Pouilly-Loché

CHABLIS

Chablis is one of the most popular names worldwide for a great variety of white and rosé wines. The original Chablis wine has a wonderfully distinctive taste that defies description.

The *grands crus* Chablis are a strong wine with a crisp, dry, gentle fruit taste, while the *premiers crus* are slightly less alcoholic and lighter in taste than the Grands Crus. Look for wines from Fiore, Moreau, and Ropiteau for top quality.

RECOMMENDED WINES:

Grands Crus:
- Bougros
- Blanchots
- Grenouilles
- Les Clos
- Les Preuses
- Valmur
- Vaudésir

Premiers Crus:
- Beugnons
- Butteaux
- Les Forêts
- Côte de Lechet
- Mont de Milieu
- Montmains
- Montée de Tonnerre
- Vaulorent

THE RHÔNE VALLEY

The Rhône vineyards, extending from Vienne to Avignon, produce some of the finest wines in southern France. The reds are velvety smooth with a deep rich flavor, while the whites are delicate but heady.

Rhône wines mature slowly, often not reaching their peak for almost a decade. Despite this, Rhône wines are the biggest bargains in French wines.

Châteauneuf-du-Pape, perhaps the most famous of Rhône wines, is a delicate blending of thirteen different grape varieties. Doctors have been recommending Châteauneuf-du-Pape to help relieve the symptoms of influenza for decades. Château Grillet is one of the best white wines of the Rhône Valley. It has a well-balanced, full-bodied dry taste. Côte Rôtie is a red Syrah grape, subtly blended with just enough white Viognier to add smoothness. Hermitage wines come from one of the oldest vineyards in France; St. Patrick is said to have first planted vines there on a visit to Gaul. Both reds and whites are produced, but the white is of exceptional interest because it is one of the longest-lived dry white wines available. Tavel exclusively produces rosé wines that enjoy a worldwide reputation. These wines do not age well and therefore should be drunk quite young, between one and five years old.

RECOMMENDED WINES:

Red

Châteauneuf-du-Pape
Cornas
Gigondas
Hermitage Rouge
Lirac Rouge
Saint-Joseph
Côte Rôtie
Côtes du Rhône

White

Hermitage Blanc

Rosé

Lirac Rosé
Tavel

Special Note: Many very good quality unknown Côtes du Rhône wines are being imported at this time at reasonable prices. Don't be afraid . . . take a chance. You can hardly go wrong with wines from this area.

CHAMPAGNE

Champagne is the most sung about, written about, romantic wine in the world. Every country produces a "Champagne," but France is the only country that legally has the right to use the name.

The quality of the wines of Champagne are due to three basic points: the unique chalky soil, the climate, and the limitless patience of the vintners. Besides the traditionally labeled

Champagne wines, there are two other important varieties produced in the chalky crevice carved out under the cities of Épernay and Reims; the Blancs de Blancs is made from white grapes, while the Blancs de Noirs is a white wine made from black grapes.

Vintage Champagnes undergo rigorous tasting by a specially appointed committee and may not be shipped before they are three years old. So beware the great buy on last year's French vintage Champagne.

Some of the more noted producers of Champagne are:

Ayala-Montebello-Duminy
Bollinger
Charles Heidsieck
De Castellane
Heidsieck Monopole
Henriot
Irroy
Krug
Lanson
Mercier
Moët et Chandon
G.H. Mumm
Perrier-Jouët
Pol Roger
Roederer
Taittinger
Veuve Clicquot
Veuve Laurent-Perrier

Sparkling wines are produced in many areas of France. A great many of the *vin mousseux,* or semi-sparkling wines, are being exported at reasonable prices. The fruity *mousseux* from the Loire and the dry sparkling wines from the Haute-Savoie are exceptionally good at substantial savings over vintage Champagne.

The physiological effects of Champagne are centuries old. Doctors have been recommending Champagne to relieve stomach distress, pain associated with hiatus hernia, rheumatism, heart disease, fever, diarrhea, and the varied complaints of the aged.

White Sparkling Wines

Clairette de Die
Seyssel (LeDuc, Boyer Brut)
St.-Péray
White Burgundy (Kriter)
Saumur
Vouvray

THE LOIRE

The picturesque Loire Valley, dotted with historic châteaux, is the home of the *vins de la Loire*. The vineyards of Anjou, Muscadet, and Vouvray produce generous quantities of white and rosé wines.

Many of the numerous fine wines of the area do not travel well due to their low alcohol level—under one percent—so the lover of fine wines must visit the vineyards personally to sample all the wonderful Loire wines.

The five major districts—Anjou, Pouilly-sur-Loire, Muscadet, Touraine, and Quincy—are world-famous for excellent wines. Although the rosé wine of the Anjou is better known, good-quality slightly sweet white and red wines are also produced. The delightfully dry white Pouilly-Fumé are made in the Pouilly-sur-Loire. This wine closely resembles the little-known dry white wine from the Quincy district. Touraine is the home of the well-known Vouvray, but other lesser-known reds, whites, and rosés of the district are exceptional values in today's wine market. Americans have discovered the dry white Muscadet wine from the district of the same name. This wine, long a favorite in France, is gaining popularity in other countries.

RECOMMENDED WINES:

Rosé

Anjou Rosé de Cabernet

Red

Bourgueil
Chinon
Saumur-Champigny

White

Bonnezeaux
Côteaux du Layon
Muscadet
Muscadet-sur-Lie
Gros Plant du Pays Nantaes
Pouilly-Fumé
Sancerre
Saumur
Savennières

ALSACE

Alsatian wines are very similar to the neighboring Rhine and Mosel vineyards but are characteristically drier, more full-bodied, and have a higher alcohol content.

Unlike the French, Alsatian wines are named after the type of grape used instead of the place of the vineyard. The almighty Riesling is heavily planted, producing a wine that is dry and fruity with only a trace of sweetness. The Sylvaner is a light fresh white that is best drunk young, an excellent refreshing summer wine selection. It is similar in taste to the Pinot Blanc but has slightly less body. The Traminer grape yields a strong spicy white, of which the best is the Gewürztraminer. The Tokay D'Alsace is on the sweet side, but with a powerful, full-bodied flavor. The Muscat D'Alsace yields a crisp, dry, fruity wine.

Alsatian wines have been successfully used in treating intestinal irritability and high blood pressure.

RECOMMENDED WINES:

Riesling
Gewürztraminer
Sylvaner

FRENCH OR CALIFORNIA? WHICH WINE?

The following chart has been developed to give a comparison between readily imported French wines and their California cousins. The wines selected are all in the $4 to $8 price range, so as not to put too much of a strain on your budget.

The chart should not be misinterpreted. The wines are not identical but only similar in style, quality, and price. Wines are listed in order of preference for each classification, but each wine is superior in its own right.

DRY WHITE WINES—LIGHT AND FRUITY

FRANCE

CALIFORNIA

Muscadet de Sèvre-et-Maine
Barre Frères 1978
La Nobleraie 1978
Réserve de la Tourmaline 1978

Chenin Blanc
Chappellet 1978
Dry Creek 1978
Foppiano 1978
Kenwood 1978

DRY WHITE WINES—FULL-BODIED

FRANCE

CALIFORNIA

Mâcon-Villages
La Grand Cheneau 1978
Les Charmes 1978

Fumé Blanc
Dry Creek 1978
Inglenook 1978
Robert Mondavi 1978

Alsatian Sylvaner 1977
Pinot Chardonnay Alexis Lichine 1977
Mouton-Cadet 1978
Saint-Véran 1977
Graves de Vayres 1978

Chardonnay
Mirassou 1978
Paul Masson Pinnacles Selection 1977
Franciscan 1978
Parducci 1978
Sonoma Vineyards River West 1978
Wente 1978

FRANCE	CALIFORNIA
Côtes de Provence Marquisat 1978	*Sauvignon Blanc*
	Sterung 1978
Moreau Blanc (non-vintage)	Callaway 1978
	Gallo (non-vintage)

RED WINES—LIGHT AND FRUITY

FRANCE	CALIFORNIA
Beaujolais-Villages 1978 & 1979	Robert Mondavi Gamay 1978
Côtes du Rhône 1977	*Gamay Beaujolais*
Corbieres (non-vintage)	Simi 1978
Côtes de Roussillon Villages (non-vintage)	Pedroncelli 1978
	Sebastiani 1978

Zinfandel
Stag's Leap Wine Cellars
Barboza 1979
Christian Brothers (non-vintage)
Sebastiani 1977
Parducci 1977
Montevina Zin Nuevo 1979

RED WINES—ROBUST, FULL-BODIED

FRANCE	CALIFORNIA
Burgundy	*Zinfandel*
Santenay-Lavières 1976	Montevina 1977
Tallot-Beaut (non-vintage)	San Martin 1976

FRANCE	CALIFORNIA
Aloxe-Corton, Senard 1976	Sutter Home 1976
Savigny-les-Beaune, Drouhin 1973	Ridge Fiddletown 1977
	Sebastiani Barbera 1972
	Inglenook Charbono 1974

153

Papagni Alicante Bouschet
1975

FRANCE

CALIFORNIA

Regional Bordeaux
Canon-Fronsac 1976
Médoc 1976
Saint-Émilion 1976
Côtes de Bourg 1976

Merlot
Château Ste. Michelle 1976
Firestone 1977
Louis Martini 1976
Monterey Vineyard Classic
Red 1977
Trefethen Eshcol Red
Fetzer Mendocino Red 1977

Bordeaux (Chateaux)
Château Moulis 196
Château Angludet 1976
Château La Cardonne 1975
Château Cos d'Estournel
1974
Château Larose-Trintaudon
1975
Château Greysac 1976
Château Fourcas-Hostein
1975

Cabernet Sauvignon
Almadén 1977
Rancho Yerba Buena 1976
Firestone 1976
Franciscan 1976
Cassayre-Forni 1976
Souverain 1976 Vintage Se-
lection

WINES OF GERMANY

Germany's northern climate provides ideal conditions for cultivating superb white wines. German wines are a delicate combination of sugar and acid balance that give them a unique crisp freshness. This balance is even more important when compared to the relatively low alcohol content (9 to 12 percent) of German wines.

The major vineyards are centered along the main rivers, the Rhine, Mosel, and Main. Although numerous grape varieties are planted, almost all the great German wines are made with the Riesling. The high-yield Sylvaner, with its slightly milder taste, and the unmistakable Gewürztraminer are also being used with more regularity as is the Müller-Thurgau, a cross between the Riesling and Sylvaner.

The German wine law of 1971 officially divided the

vineyards into eleven wine-making districts: Ahr, Baden, Nahe, Rheinhessen, Franken, Rheinpfalz, Ruwer, Rheingau, Mittelrhein, Hessiche Bergstrasse, and Würtemberg.

Quality German wine is definitely worth the effort to find and the standardized labeling law makes understanding the label much simpler. The best wines are classed *Qualitätswein mit Prädikat* ("quality wine with special attribute"). These wines must state their origin: Mosel, Saar, Rheinpfalz, Nahe, etc. As in France, estate-bottled wine will denote *original abfüllung* or *Erzeugerabfüllung, aus eigenem Lesegut* (bottled by the producer from his own grapes). More important to the consumer are the "special attributes" that are based on the *Öchsle* (sweetness) scale:

Kabinett—	75 öchsle; driest, without added sugar
Spätlese—	80 öchsle; late harvest, flavorful, fruity
Auslese—	90 öchsle; finest selection of grapes, pressed separately
Beerenauslese—	120 öchsle; selected berry harvest
Trockenbeerenauslese—	150 öchsle; selected individual dry berries, very sweet

German wines have been used to treat a wide spectrum of disease since the Romans settled along the banks of the Rhine. Rhine wines are being successfully used in appetite control, while Mosel wines help relieve constipation, and Ahr, Saar, and Nahe are receiving increased attention in relation to cholesterol reduction.

While it would be impossible to list all the great imported German wines, I will attempt to recommend several in each district that are outstanding for both quality and price and, in addition, list the outstanding vineyards so that you can easily recognize top-quality imports.

THE RHEINGAU

The more than 7,000 acres of grapes in the Rheingau area are almost exclusively planted for white wine. The Rheingau has always been considered one of the top-quality wine areas of Germany. It gives the consumer an enormous variety of flavors ranging from spicy to smooth and elegant. The 150 acres of red wine grapes grown in the Rheingau at Assmannhausen provide some of Germany's best.

RECOMMENDED WINES:

Erbacher Marcobrunn Kabinett, von Simmern
Hattenheimer Nussbrunnen Kabinett, von Simmern
Rüdesheimer Berg Schlossberg Kabinett, von Schorlemer
Rauenthaler Baiken Kabinett, Graf Eltz
Schloss Johannisberg Orange Seal Kabinett
Schloss Vollrads Blue/Gold Kabinett
Furstlich Löwenstein, Kabinett, Hallgartener Schönhell
Hochheimer Domdechaney, Kabinett
Schloss Groenesteyn, Rüdesheimer Berg Rottland, Kabinett

OUTSTANDING VINEYARDS:

Town	Vineyard
Eltville	Sonnenberg, Langenstück
Erbach	Marcobrunner, Siegelsberg, Steinmorgen
Geisenheim	Rothenberg
Hallgarten	Deutelsberg, Schönhell
Hattenhein	Steinberg, Nussbrunnen, Wisselbrunnen
Hochheim	Domdechaney
Johannisberg	Schloss Johannisberg, Hölle, Klaus
Kiedrich	Gräfenberg, Wasserrose
Oestrich	Eiserberg

Rauenthal	Baiken, Gehrn
Rüdesheim	Berg Bronnen, Berg Lay, Berg Burgweg, Berg Rottland
Winkel	Schloss Vollrads

RHEINHESSEN

The Rheinhessen, or Hesse, as it is more commonly called throughout the world, produces popular soft light wines. The town of Nierstein is the home of the finest Rheinhessen wines. More than half a million gallons of Niersteiner wine are produced annually.

RECOMMENDED WINES:

Niersteiner Hipping Kabinett, Franz Karl Schmitt
Niersteiner Orbel Kabinett, Franz Karl Schmitt
Niersteiner Auflangen Kabinett, Reinhold Senfter
Oppenheimer Sackträger Kabinett, Reinhold Senfter

OUTSTANDING VINEYARDS:

Town	*Vineyard*
Bingen	Eiselberg, Rochusberg, Rosengarten
Bodenheim	Hock, Ebersberg
Dienheim	Falkenberg
Nackenheim	Engelsberg, Rothenberg
Nierstein	collective names are now being used—the best-known names that produce a remarkably good wine are: Glöck, Hipping, Kranzberg, Orbel, Oelberg, Pettenthal,

	Rosenberg, Rehbach, and Zehnmorgen
Oppenheim	Kreuz, Sackträger

RHEINPFALZ (THE PALATINATE)

Germany's largest wine-producing region covers almost 40,-000 acres, yielding 20 million gallons of wine annually. Unfortunately, not all of this wine is of top quality, having a distinctly earthy taste that is harsh. The best wines of the region are produced in the tiny area known as the Mittelhaardt. Many of the great wines of the Pfalz are produced in the town of Deidesheim by three outstanding vintners: Bürklin-Wolf, von Buhl, and Bassermann-Jordan.

RECOMMENDED WINES:

Diedesheimer Hohenmorgen Kabinett, Dr. Bürklin-Wolf
Forster Kirchenstück Kabinett, von Buhl
Forster Jesuitengarten Kabinett, Bassermann-Jordan
Ruppertsberger Gaisböhl Kabinett, Dr. Bürklin-Wolf

OUTSTANDING VINEYARDS:

Town	Vineyard
Bad Dürkheim	Michelsberg
Deidesheim	Herrgottsacker, Grainhübel, Leinhöhle
Forst	Kirchenstück, Jesuitengarten Freudstück
Königsbach	Bender, Idig
Ruppertsberg	Hoheberg
Wachenheim	Gerümpel, Bächel

MOSEL-SAAR-RUWER

The picturesque Mosel flows northward from its source in France, passing quaint towns and great vineyards.

Many of the Mosel wines are equally as good as the best produced in the neighboring Rheinland, although totally different in character.

Some of the best Mosel wines come from the storybook town of Bernkastel, more specifically the southern slope called the Doktorberg. While other excellent wines are produced in Wehlen, Graahen, Piesport, and Zeltingen, nothing quite compares to the Bernkasteler Doktor.

Mosels are delightful wines, low in alcohol with a delicate, fragrant, full Riesling bouquet.

The Mosel's two confluents, the Saar and the Ruwer, produce excellent wines. The best Saar wines come from the Scharzhofberger, where the winegrowers use oil burners to thwart untimely frosts.

Although the Ruwer is only a rivulet, two of its wine districts, the Eitelsbacher and Maximin Grünhaus, have gained an international reputation. Ruwer wines are light, sometimes naturally sparkling, and rival the best of the Mosels.

RECOMMENDED WINES:

Urziger Würzgarten Kabinett, Jos. Beeres
Josephshöfer Kabinett, von Kesselstatt
Bernkasteler Schlossberg Kabinett, Wwe. Dr. Thanisch
Piesporter Goldtröpfchen Kabinett, Viet
Maximin Grünhauser Herrenberg Kabinett, C. von Schubert
Scharzhofberger Kabinett, Egon Müller
Graacher Himmelreich Kabinett, J.J. Prüm
Avelsbacher Altenberg Kabinett, Hohe Domkirche
Oberemmeler Scharzberg Kabinett, Reichsgraf von Kesselstatt

OUTSTANDING VINEYARDS:

Town	Vineyard
Bernkastel	Doktor, Lay

Brauneberg	Juffer, Falkenberg
Erden	Treppchen. Prälat
Graach	Josephshöfer, Himmelreich
Piesport	Goldtröpfchen, Lay
Ürzig	Würzgarten, Schwarzlay
Wehlen	Sonnenuhr, Nonnenberg
Zeltingen	Himmelreich, Schlossberg

WINES OF ITALY

Due to Italy's diverse climate, soil consistency, and grape varieties, a wide selection of wines ranging from everyday table wines to great vintages is produced.

Italy, land of wine, produces almost a billion and a half gallons of wine annually. Italians are born wine-lovers, with a per capita consumption of nearly thirty gallons a year.

The majority of Italian wines are ordinary and undistinguished, but a good vintage Verdicchio or Soave is very enjoyable. Although vineyards are scattered everywhere throughout the country, the best-quality wines are produced in northern and central Italy.

Italian wine labeling is reliable, wines being named after the grape variety, town of origin, or production district. This is the result of the establishment of government controls in 1963 and recent further moves to correct Italian wine producers' nonchalant attitude toward nomenclature. The following classifications have helped the consumer develop a more serious attitude toward Italian wines:

1. *Denominazione di origine simplice* denotes ordinary wine grown in specified areas. It is not a quality rating.
2. *Denominazione di origine controllata* applies to wines that have passed controlled standards of testing.
3. *Denominazione di origine controllata e garantita* denotes only the finest wines that meet not only quality but price standards imposed by the government.

160

Besides the above government controls, voluntary controls are exercised by the National Institute for the Inspection of Identification of Origin (*Institutione del comitato nazionale per la tutela delle denominazione di origine*). The Institute awards a red seal to Italian wines that are authorized for export.

To understand Italian wines, it is important to know the regions where they are produced.

REGION	WINE TYPE
Abruzzi	Red: Montepulciano White: Trebbiano
Calabria	Red: Cirò di Calabria Sweet White: Greco di Gerace
Campania	Red: Falerno White: Lacrima Christi Falerno
Emilia-Romagna	Red: Lambrusco Sangiovese
Latium	Dry White: Frascati Est! Est! Est!
Lombardy	Red: Sassella Grumello Fracia Inferno Rosé: Chiaretto
Lucania	Red: Anglianico del Vulture
Piedmont	Red: Barolo Barbaresco Barbera Freisa Gattinara Grignolino Nebbiolo

	Sweet-Sparkling: Asti Spumante

Tuscany	Red: Chianti Sweet white: Vin Santo

Umbria	White: Orvieto (dry/sweet)

Sardinia	Moscato Sweet/fortified White: Moscato Malvasia

Sicily	Red: Faro
	    Corvo di Casteldaccia
	      Etna
	White: Mamertino
	    Corvo di Casteldaccia
	      Etna

The best of the region is the superb Marsala.

Veneto	Red: Bardolino
	    Valpolicella
	    Valpantena
	White: Soave

CHAPTER TWELVE

AMERICAN WINES

American wine is worthy of attention, and a good many people are now beginning to give it the attention it deserves, but there is still a need for more accurate and basic taste information on it. The majority of Americans are probably unfamiliar with any but the largest vineyards, whose advertising floods the market. They react with surprise at learning that some of the best American wines are produced in New York State.

There are many excellent books on the subject of wine production and quality control, but very few come out and tell the consumer directly what he really wants to know and is very often embarrassed to ask—what the wine tastes like.

In this chapter I have given the reader an up-to-date and simple taste description for a cross section of American wines. It should be much more helpful than most rating scales, which I feel are not only misleading, but not very informative for the average buyer.

I hope, through tasting, the reader will discover the happy surprises that American wines have to offer.

THE WINES OF CALIFORNIA and NEW YORK

RED WINES

WINE NAME	DESCRIPTION
Almadén Vineyards Los Gatos, CA	
California Barbera	Fruity, semi-dry, moderate acid balance
California Burgundy	Semi-dry, pleasing tart edge, shows good blending of youth and maturity
California Original	Fresh, fruity bouquet with moderate acid balance
California Mountain Red Burgundy	Somber, dignified, muted fruit taste
California Mountain Red Claret	Medium red, slightly coarse, hearty taste with a trace of bitterness
California Zinfandel	Slightly rough, musty, sharp, fruity taste—excellent companion for hot, spicy food
Beaulieu Vineyard Rutherford, CA	
Beaulieu Vineyard Napa Valley Burgundy	Rich, heady, well-rounded fruity taste
Beaumont Pinot Noir Private Reserve Cabernet Sauvignon	Dry, fresh, pleasing; a remarkable wine, well rounded

Beringer Vineyards Los
Hermanos Vineyards
St. Helena, CA

California Barenblut	Dry, light, enjoyable
California Grignolino	Very unusual fruity taste with a slightly spicy after-taste—very pleasant
California Zinfandel	Slightly heavy wine with a pleasant fruit and acid balance
North Coast Burgundy	Light, fresh, fruity wine

Boordy Vineyards
Penn Yan, NY

Boordy Vineyards Pinard	Light, fresh, fruity
Boordy Vineyards Red Wine	Unusual flavor, slightly stuffy

The Brotherhood Corpora-
tion, Washingtonville, NY
(America's oldest winery)

Holiday	A special red—spicy, with herbs
Burgundy	Dry, full flavor

Beuna Vista Winery
and Vineyards
Sonoma, CA

Buena Vista Zinfandel	A remarkable wine, mature, fruity

CC Vineyard
Winery
Ceres, CA

| CC Vineyard California Burgundy | Moderately dry, fresh, fruity flavor |

Lodi Vintners
Bottler: Carnot Vintners
Acampo, CA

| Château Vin Burgundy | Enjoyable, slightly sweet taste—good with meals |

Cappella Wineries
San Francisco, CA

| Cappella Red Table Wine | Slightly sweet/tart taste |

Carlo Rossi Vineyards
Modesto, CA

| Carlo Rossi's Red Mountain California Light Chanti | Simple, slightly sweet, refreshing taste |

Lee Pashick
Napa.
Calistoga, CA

| Château Montelena Cabernet Sauvignon | Beautifully balanced, powerful |

The Christian Bros.
Napa, CA

| Christian Brothers Select California Burgundy | Dry, mature, fruity taste, slightly tart |

Cabernet Sauvignon

Brother Timothy Zinfandel

Cresta Blanca
Winery
San Francisco, CA

Cresta Blanca Mendocino Gamay Beaujolais	Light, very dry, crisp taste
Cresta Blanca Mendocino Zinfandel	Full body, zesty, slightly tart fruit taste

B. Cribari & Sons
San Francisco, CA

Famiglia Cribari California Cabernet Sauvignon	Medium dry, well-rounded, fruity flavor.
Famiglia Cribari California Vino Rosso da Pranzo	Light, simple fruity—good flavor.

Delicato Vineyards
Manteca, CA

Delicato Especially Selected California Burgundy	Dry taste of matured fruit, more like a Bordeaux than a Burgundy

Fetzer Vineyards
Redwood Valley, CA

Fetzer Vineyards Lake Country Zinfandel	Well-rounded, mellow fruity taste

Freemark Abbey Winery
St. Helena
Napa, CA

Cabernet Sauvignon	Outclasses all competitors by a mile—powerful
Cabernet Bosche	Superb—no comparison

Ernest & Julio Gallo Winery
Modesto, CA

California Barbera	Very dry, lively
California Burgundy	Mild, fruity
Hearty Burgundy	Fruity with a slight sweet/sour tartness
Ruby Cabernet	Potent, almost dry fresh taste
California Zinfandel	Light, slightly bitter taste

Giumarra Vineyards
Edison, CA

Giumarra Classic California Burgundy	Semi-dry, fruity, tart

California Growers
Winery, Inc.
San Francisco, CA

California Burgundy	Slightly sweet, fully ripe, mature flavor
California Cabernet Sauvignon	Slightly harsh taste
California Ruby Cabernet	Slightly sweet
California Zinfandel	Agreeable taste

Heitz Wine Cellars
St. Helena, CA

Heitz Cellars Cabernet Sauvignon	Richness, depth—superb

Inglenook Vineyards
San Francisco, CA

California Navalle Burgundy	Dry, vigorous, ripe grape flavor
California Navalle Claret	Mature, semi-dry, fruity
California Navalle Ruby Cabernet	Pleasing taste—clean, straightforward
California Navalle Zinfandel	Spicy, fruity
North Coast Counties Vintage Burgundy	Smooth, dry, mature, fruity

Italian Swiss Colony
Asti, CA

California Barbera	Hardy, bracing, excellent table wine
California Burgundy	Refreshing, slightly biting, fruity
California Cabernet Sauvignon	Simple, young, biting
California Chianti	Fruity, slightly sweet
California Ruby Cabernet	Refreshing, with vigor and character
California Zinfandel	Fruity, spicy, interesting

F. Korbel & Bros.
Guerneville, CA

Korbel California Burgundy — Well-balanced, fruity, wonderfully tart edge

Korbel California Zinfandel — Dry, fruity, spicy with vigor

Charles Krug Winery
St. Helena, CA

Napa Valley Vintage Burgundy — Spicy, herbal, fresh, invigorating

Napa Valley Claret — Slightly sour

Napa Valley Gamay Beaujolais — Light, dry, fruity

Cabernet Sauvignon — Well-balanced, good character

M. LaMont Vineyards
LaMont, CA

California Burgundy — Dry, fruity, slightly astringent

California Cabernet — Dry, smooth, refreshing

California Zinfandel — Dry, fruity, good acid balance

Los Hermanos Vineyards
St. Helena, CA

California Burgundy — Interesting sweet/sour taste

California Gamay Beaujolais	Fruity, touch of sweetness
California Zinfandel	Refreshing, fruity

Louis M. Martini
St. Helena, CA

California Burgundy	Dry, rich, fruity
California Mountain Chianti	Simple, fruity, bracing
California Mountain Claret	Light, refreshing
California Mountain Red Wine	Dry, slightly spicy, tart edge
California Zinfandel	Well-balanced, fruity and spicy

Paul Masson Vineyards
Saratoga, CA

Baroque	Rich, smooth, well-balanced
California Burgundy	Dry, astringent
California Gamay Beaujolais	Light, dry, slightly fruity, spicy
California Petite Sirah	Pleasant, exotic, fruity
California Pinot Noir	Dry, fresh—pleasing flavor on the thin side
California Zinfandel	Pleasant, well-balanced, refreshing

Rubion	Light, dry, slightly tart

Mirassou Vineyards
San Jose, CA

Mirassou Santa Clara Burgundy	Rich, full, fruity

C. Mondavi & Sons
St. Helena, CA

California Select Barberone	Masculine, fruity, well-rounded
California Select Burgundy	Subdued, fresh, fruity
California Select Chianti	Refreshing, robust, fruity
California Select Claret	Dry, forceful, mature fruity taste
California Select Zinfandel	Dry, fruity, mature but light

Robert Mondavi Winery
Oakville, CA

Robert Mondavi California Red Table Wine	Fruity, good balance, a little thin
Cabernet Sauvignon	Well-rounded, good flavor
Pinot Noir	Dry, fresh, pleasing

Novitiate of Los Gatos
Los Gatos, CA

Novitiate California Burgundy	Semi-dry, fruity, mature, masculine

**Papagni Vineyards
Madera, CA**

California Barbera	Dry, fresh, spicy
California Zinfandel	Energetic, fresh, tart

**Parducci Wine Cellars
Ukiah, CA**

Parducci California Vintage Burgundy	Moderately dry, mild, fruity

**San Martin Vineyards Co., Inc.
San Martin, CA**

San Martin Santa Clara Valley Burgundy	Dry, zesty, fruity

**Sebastiani Vineyards
Sonoma, CA**

North Coast Counties Burgundy	Dry, fresh, fruity
North Coast Counties Chianti	Energetic, refreshing, full-bodied
Northern California Burgundy	Dry, mature, quiet
Northern California Mountain Cabernet Sauvignon	Mild, fruity, refreshing, mature

Zinfandel   Nothing spectacular—
                                   slightly flat

Robert Setrakian Vineyards
Yettem, CA

   Setrakian Mountain Red   Rich, elegant, smooth
   Burgundy

Sonoma Vineyards
Windsor, CA

   Sonoma County Gamay   Fresh, engaging, fruity
   Beaujolais

   Sonoma Vineyards Zin-   Taste of excellent breeding,
   fandel   enjoyable

Souverain Cellars
Geyserville, CA

   Souverain of Alexander   Dry, medium body, fruity
   Valley North Coast Bur-
   gundy

   Souverain of Alexander   Dry, light, ripe, full of fruit
   Valley Sonoma Zinfandel

Sterling Vineyards
Calistoga, CA

   Sterling Napa Valley Red   Fresh, clean taste, full of
   Wine   fruit

The Taylor Wine Co., Inc.
Hammondsport, NY

   Taylor Lake Country Red   Sweet, grapey

Weibel Champagne
Vineyards
Mission San Jose, CA

    Weibel California Classic   Moderately dry, fruity, zesty
    Burgundy

Wente Brothers
Livermore, CA

    Wente Brothers Zinfandel   Slightly sweet, fruity

Winemasters' Guild
San Francisco, CA

    California Cabernet Sau-   Dry, light, fruity
    vignon

    California Mountain   Semi-dry, fresh, fruity
    Burgundy

    California Ruby   Thin, stale, negative back-
    Cabernet   taste

    California Zinfandel   Rich, full, fruity

WHITE WINES

WINE NAME	DESCRIPTION

Almadén Vineyards
Los Gatos, CA

    California Chablis   Slightly flat, dry, austere,
    bitter taste

    California French Colom-   Pleasant, well-rounded,
    bard   fruity

California Mountain Rhine	Light, hint of sweetness—appealing
California Mountain White Chablis	Dry, light
California Mountain White Sauterne	Thin, light, sour taste

Beaulieu Vineyard
Rutherford, CA

Bealulieu Vineyard Napa Valley Chablis	Slightly sweet, fruity

Beringer Vineyards/Los
Hermanos Vineyards
St. Helena, CA

California Traubengold	Fresh, clean, fruity
North Coast Chablis	Light, refreshing, unusual lemon flavor
North Coast Chenin Blanc	Light, sweet, fruity, honey-flavored
North Coast Grey Riesling	Moderately dry, fresh, fruity

J.E.J. Bronco Winery
Ceres, CA

Bronco California Chablis	Healthy, lightly sweet, moderately fruity

The Brotherhood Corporation
Washingtonille, NY

Chablis   Light, dry, refreshing

Buena Vista Winery and
Vineyards
Sonoma, CA

   Buena Vista Sonoma Cha-   Semi-dry, clean, fruity
   blis

Carlo Rossi Vineyards
Modesto, CA

   Red Mountain California   Semi-dry, fresh, fruity, light
   Chablis

   Red Mountain California   Sweetish, slightly flat taste
   Rhine

The Christian Bros.
Napa, CA

   Château LaSalle   Well-rounded, fruity,
                                fragrant

   Select California Chablis   Rich, fruity, smooth

   Select California Haut   Sweet, ripe grape flavor
   Sauterne

   Select California Sauterne   Full, fruity, aromatic

Cresta Blanca Winery
San Francisco, CA

   California Blanc de Blanc   Sweet, mature, delicate

   California Chenin Blanc   Fruity, light, mature

| California French Colombard | Light, fruity sweetness |
| California Mountain Chablis | Slightly brash, aggressive |

B. Cribari & Sons
San Francisco, CA

California Mountain Chablis	A very real, serious Chablis
California Sauterne	Semi-dry, mildly fruity
California Vino Blanco da Pranzo	Mild, fruity, sweet

Delicato Vineyards
Manteca, CA

Especially Selected California Chablis Blanc	Semi-dry, masculine, with a slight bitterness
Especially Selected California Chenin Blanc	Mild fruit
Especially Selected California Rhine	Simple, clean, fruity

Fetzer Vineyards
Redwood Valley, CA

| Fetzer Vineyards Mendocino Premium White | Slightly sweet, light, clean |

Ernest & Julio Gallo Winery
Modesto, CA

California Chablis Blanc	Nicely balanced, gentle, light
California Chenin Blanc	Semi-dry, fresh, fruity
California French Colombard	Modest, undistinguished
California Rhine Garten	Light, slightly sweet, soft
California Rhine Wine	Aromatic, sweet, on the heavy side—pleasant
California Riesling	Fresh, fruity, pleasant

California Growers Winery, Inc.
San Francisco, CA

| California Chenin Blanc | Light, dry, slightly bitter |
| California French Colombard | Thin, flat, slightly sweet |

Guasti Vintners
Delano, CA

| Guasti California French Colombard | Light, delicately sweet, fruity |

Inglenook Vineyards
San Francisco, CA

Navalle Chablis	Slightly sweet, light, clean
California Navalle Chenin Blanc	Fruity, slightly sweet
California Navalle Rhine	Slightly flat and sweet

North Coast Counties Vintage Chablis	Light, dry, refreshing

Italian Swiss Colony
Asti, CA

California Chablis	Fruity, well-balanced, slightly sweet
California Chenin Blanc	Fruity, slightly sweet, spicy, well-balanced
California French Colombard	Fresh, fruity, pleasantly tart
California Rhine	Fruity, slightly flat
California Sauterne	Fruity, moderately sweet, velvety
Emerald Chablis	Syrupy taste
Gold Chablis	Extremely fruity, slightly sweet honey flavor

F. Korbel & Bros.
Guerneville, CA

California Chablis	Moderately dry, light
California Chenin Blanc	Dry, cheerful, pleasant
California Grey Riesling	Slightly bitter, woody taste

Charles Krug Winery
St. Helena, CA

Napa Valley Chablis	Fruity, good balance
Napa Valley Chenin Blanc	Dry, light, ripe, fruity
Napa Valley Dry Sauterne	Slightly fruity

180

Napa Valley Grey Rielsing	Slightly sweet, clean, feminine wine
Napa Valley Traminer	Dry, crisp, herbal

M. LaMont Vineyards
LaMont, CA

California Chablis	Simple, ordinary
California French Colombard	Unexceptional

Los Hermanós Vineyards
St. Helena, CA

California Chablis	Fruity, slightly sweet, enjoyable
California Chardonnay	Dry, zesty, tart, fruity
California Chenin Blanc	Mildly fruity, sweet
California Johannisberg Riesling	Semi-dry, crisp, fruity, pleasing

Louis M. Martini
St. Helena, CA

California Mountain Chablis	Refreshing sweet/sour mixture
California Mountain Dry Sauterne	Mediocre, restrained
California Mountain White Chablis	Dry, light, pleasingly tart

Paul Masson Vineyards
Saratoga, CA

California Chablis	Refreshing, nicely balanced
California Chenin Blanc	Agreeable
California Rhine	Not sweet/not dry but pleasingly refreshing
California Sauterne Château Masson	Heavy, syrupy sweet
Emerald Dry White Table Wine	Well-balanced, fruity, bracing, only slightly sweet
Rhine Castle	Thick, sweet—good dessert wine

C. Mondavi & Sons
St. Helena, CA

California Select Chablis	Light, modestly sweet
California Select Dry Sauterne	Semi-dry, fruity, pleasant
California Select Rhine	Spicy, good balance, not sweet or tart—just right

Robert Mondavi Winery
Oakville, CA

Robert Mondavi California White Table Wine	Refreshing, light, fruity

Novitiate of Los Gatos
Los Gatos, CA

Novitiate California Pinot Blanc	Mature, refined

Papagni Vineyards
Madera, CA

Angelo Papagni California Muscat Alexandria	Rich, ripe, fruity

Parducci Wine Cellars
Ukiah, CA

Parducci Mendocino Country French Colombard	Well-balanced, mildly sweet

J. Pedroncelli Winery
Geyserville, CA

Pedroncelli Sonoma White Wine	Soft, fruity, slightly sweet

Petri Wineries
San Francisco, CA

California Chablis Blanc	Delicate, semi-sweet, fruity
California Sauterne	Semi-dry, fruity, lively

Sebastiani Vineyards
Sonoma, CA

North Coast Counties Chablis	Thin, slightly flat with a bitter aftertaste
North Coast Counties Green Hungarian	Well-balanced, slightly sweet, fruity

Northern California
Chenin Blanc

Slightly sweet, fruity

Northern California
Mountain Pinot Chardon-
nay

Semi-dry, sweet/sour, well-
balanced fruitiness

Souverain Cellars
Geyserville, CA

Souverain of Alexander
Valley North Coast Dry
Chenin Blanc

Dry, reserved, full-bodied

Sterling Vineyards
Calistoga, CA

Sterling Napa Valley
White Table Wine

Well-balanced, fruity

Weibel Champagne Vine-
yards
Mission San Jose, CA

California Classic Chablis

Fresh, slightly sweet, well-
balanced

California Green Hun-
garian

Sweet, heavy, flowery

California Hoffberg
May Wine

Smooth, herbal, well-
balanced

Wente Brothers
Livermore, CA

California Chablis

Well-balanced, pleasing—
touch of sweetness.

| California Grey Riesling | Refreshing |

Winemasters' Guild
San Francisco, CA

California Chenin Blanc	Mildly sweet, fruity, pleasant
California French Colombard	Spicy, refreshing
California Johannisberg Riesling	Slightly sweet, inviting, refreshing
California Mountain Chablis	Fruity, tart, refreshing
Gewürztraminer	Fruity, spicy, nice

WINERY PUBLICATIONS

Many wineries publish newsletters that detail specific wine production methods and discuss future wine trends. For additional information about these newsletters, write to the individual vineyards:

The Grapevine, Buena Vista Winery, P. O. Box 182, Sonoma, CA 95476.

News from the Peak, Geyser Peak Winery, 4340 Redwood Highway, Suite 220, San Rafael, CA 94903.

Winemasters' News, Guild Wineries and Distilleries, 500 Sansome St., San Francisco, CA 94111.

Latest Press, Mirassou Vineyards, Rt. 3, Box 344, San Jose, CA 95121.

Sebastiani Vineyards, Inc., P. O. Box AA, 389 Fourth St. E., Sonoma, CA 95476.

Vineyard Vignettes, Concannon Vineyard, P.O. Box 432, Livermore, CA 95452.

Bottles and Bins, Charles Krug Winery, P.O. Box 191, St. Helena CA 94574.

Papagni Press, Papagni Vineyards, 31754 Ave. 9, Madera, CA 93637.

Hans Kornell Champagne Newsletter, Hanns Kornell Champagne Cellars, Box 249, St. Helena, CA 94574.

Inglenook Notes, Inglenook Vineyards, P.O. Box 19, Rutherford, CA 94573.

Winemaker Notes, The Monterey Vineyard, Box 780, Gonzales, CA 93926.

The Woodinville Press, Ste. Michelle Vintners, P.O. Box 1976, Woodinville, WA 98072.

For additional information on California wines, write to The Wine Institute, 165 Post Street, San Francisco, CA 94108. The Institute offers a wide variety of interesting material that includes a free touring guide of the California wineries, "California's Wine Wonderland," and an extremely interesting "Wine Study Course" is also offered free.

Information and publications on the Eastern and Midwestern wineries can be obtained from The American Wine Society, 4218 Rosewold Ave., Royal Oak, MI 48073. The *American Wine Society Journal* is a quarterly publication of the society and is available for a subscription price of $12.50.

Friends of Wine, *Les Amis du Vin,* is a national association divided into local chapters that meet for lectures, dinners, and wine tasting. For more information on joining or subscribing to their bimonthly magazine (cost $9 yearly), write to the association at 2302 Perkins Place, Silver Springs, MD 20910.

TOURING THE WINERIES

Organizing a tour of the wineries is often as much hard work as fun. The Wine Institute publishes several valuable booklets. In addition, the Vintage Image, 1335 Main St., St. Helena, CA 94544, privately publishes three touring booklets: "Sonoma Mendocino Wine Tour," "Napa Valley Wine Tour," and "Central Coast Wine Tour." Each booklet costs $5.95 and is well worth the price.

For information on the New York State wineries, send twenty-five cents for the "New York State Wines and Champagnes and Guide to Wineries," to the New York State Department of Agriculture and Markets, Bldg. 8, State Campus, Albany, NY 12235.

Most of the large wineries operate scheduled tours, but appointments are necessary at smaller family-operated wineries. The timing of your visit is extremely important. The harvest season brings substantial crowds and long lines that distract from the enjoyment of the vineyards.

The majority of large vineyards have well-organized tours that demonstrate how wine is made and even sell boxed lunches and wine for picnicking on the grounds. But the tasting room seems to be the undisputed success of the tour, and tolerance may limit the number of wineries visited per day.

APPENDIX A

ALCOHOL AND DRUG INTERACTIONS: A WORD TO THE WISE

Antihistamines should be classified as sedatives, for when combined with alcohol, a marked increase in the sedative effect is noticed. It is extremely dangerous to drive or operate any machine while combining alcohol and antihistamines. If you want to be safe, never mix antihistamine medication with alcohol, as the individual exaggerated responses vary.

Epileptics taking the anticonvulsant drug Dilantin should understand that alcohol increases the normal rate of metabolizing the drug, and seizures may occur after prolonged heavy drinking episodes.

Many of the common antidepressant drugs prescribed today, such as Aventyl, Elavil, Norpramin, Sinequan, and Tofranil, when combined with alcohol only intensify the depressant effect that alcohol has on the central nervous system. Many people are killed each year while trying to drive or operate complicated machinery while under the influence of an antidepressant drug and alcohol. Medical research also indicates that this dangerous combination may cause increased liver difficulty while lowering the seizure threshold.

The monoamine-oxidase inhibitors are another type of common antidepressant drug that includes such preparations as Eutonyl, Marplan, and Mardil. They also do not combine well with alcohol because they tend to slow down the actual metabolism of the alcohol in the body and strengthen the central nervous system depressant effect. Many patients using this type of antidepressant drug and alcohol, especially beer and Chianti wine, experience sudden rapid blood pressure increases, and Antabuse-type reactions have been experienced. (Disulfuram or Antabuse is commonly used in a program to promote alcohol abstinence, and when combined with alcohol produces extremely unpleasant side effects such as nausea, vomiting, painful throbbing in the head and sick, extreme headaches, difficulty in breathing, and hot flushing of the skin.)

The phenothiazines are the major tranquilizers and the antidepressant drugs Compazine, Mellaril, Repose, Tindal, and Thorazine are widely prescribed to treat psychotic patients. When combined with alcohol, these drugs produce a depression of the respiratory control centers that can lead to death. Phenothiazines tend to lower the body's normal seizure threshold and when combined with large quantities of alcohol increase the risk of convulsions and can intensify drug-induced irregular heart rhythms and low blood pressure.

The most widely prescribed group of minor tranquilizers and barbiturates produce effects similar to those of alcohol, and when combined cause bizarre effects on the central nervous system that include impaired judgment, decreased alertness, imparied motor coordination and manual dexterity, as well as sudden and dangerous lowering of the blood pressure.

Valium, one of the most widely prescribed tranquilizers in the world, in many cases affects the body's tolerance of alcohol. The combined effect can cause heart, circulatory, and respiratory collapse.

Chloral hydrate—better known as *the* ingredient in a "Mickey Finn"—combined with alcohol can cause respiratory arrest and death.

When stimulants such as amphetamines and caffeine are combined with alcohol, the body appears more alert, but the alcohol has not actually relieved the depressant effect or improved motor functions. Each person's response to these drugs differs widely, and bizarre effects on the cardiovascular system have been experienced, including hypertension, rapid heartbeat, and convulsions.

Narcotic drugs such as Dilaudid, Demerol, and Darvon work as depressants of the central nervous system, and their effect is greatly increased by alcohol. The combination can effectively depress the center of breathing control until breathing stops completely.

If you are taking an antihypertension drug—for example, Aldomet, Apresoline, Dralzine, Esimil, Ismelin, or Reserpine—there is no clinical evidence that combination with alcohol produces unhealthy side effects; alcohol may cause an increase in the drug's effectiveness in controlling high blood pressure.

Each patient's response to a medication is different, and many people never consider alcohol as a common denominator in drug-related reactions. Ask your physician before including wine or any form of alcohol in your diet while taking a specific medication. The following chart indicates common medications and complications when combined with alcohol.

ALCOHOL AND DRUG INTERACTIONS

Drugs	*Adverse Effects with Alcohol*
Insulin, or all antidiabetic medication	Exaggerated insulin response, hypoglycemia
Antihistamines, hay fever medication, over-the-counter cold medications: Contac, Coricidin, Benadryl, etc.	Increased sedative reaction
Non-narcotic analgesics: salicylates, aspirin	Acute stomach irritation, increased gastric bleeding
Narcotic analgesics: Demerol, morphine, Methadone, Codeine	Depressed brain activity, possible respiratory arrest
Antihypertensives: Mecalymine, Reserpine, Deserpidine, Quanethidine, etc.	Increased sedative and hypertensive action
Amphetamines: caffeine, and other central nervous system stimulants	Euphoric, false sense of security

Sedatives, bromides, barbiturates and non-barbiturates	Extreme sedation, respiratory arrest, coma, and death Antidepressants: Doxepin,
Tranquilizers	Extreme sedation, severely impaired motor skills
Anticonvulsant: Dilantin	Decreased effectiveness
Antidepressants: Doxepin, Imipramine, monoamine-oxidase inhibitors, etc.	Increased sedative effect; Chianti wines should definitely be avoided
Antialcohol: Antabuse, Calcium Carbamide	Headache, nausea, vomiting, high blood pressure, palpitations, and occasionally death
Diuretics: Quinethazone, Thiazide, Furosemide, etc.	Hypotension
Anticoagulants: Phenindamine, Acenocoumaral	Decreased effectiveness
Vitamins, A, B, B_{12}, D, E, folic acid, K	Decreased absorption with heavy alcohol intake

APPENDIX B

CALORIC CONTENT OF MAJOR WINE TYPES

Wine	Cal./ 100cc	Cal./ oz.	Typical serving (oz.)	Cal./ typical serving
Red Table Wines:				
Barbera	81.3	24.4	4	97.6
Burgundy	80.2	24.1	4	96.4
Cabernet	82.8	24.8	4	99.2
Chianti	81.8	24.5	4	98.0
Claret	79.8	23.9	4	95.6
Zinfandel	81.8	24.5	4	98.0
Rosé Table Wines	78.3	23.5	4	94.0
White Table Wines:				
Chablis	73.8	22.1	4	88.4
Champagne	82.5	24.8	4	99.2
Rhine	76.7	23.0	4	92.0
Riesling	74.8	22.4	4	89.6
Dry sauterne	74.8	22.4	4	89.6
Sauterne	77.2	23.2	4	92.8
Sweet sauterne	87.1	26.1	4	104.4
Apéritif and Dessert Wines:				
Red port	161.3	48.4	2	96.8
White port	150.0	45.0	2	90.0
Muscatel	163.2	49.0	2	98.0
Dry sherry	130.1	39.0	2	78.0
Sweet sherry	152.7	45.8	2	91.6
Dry vermouth	113.2	34.0	3	102.0
Sweet vermouth	150.4	45.1	3	135.3

From Leake, C.D., and Silverman, M. *Alcoholic Beverages in Clinical Medicine*. Chicago: Year Book Medical Publishers, Inc., 1966.

APPENDIX C

CALORIE COUNTER

FRUIT	CALORIES
Apple	
Baked, 1 medium	188
Fresh, 1 medium	70
Juice, 1 cup	120
Applesauce	
Sweetened, ½ cup	115
Unsweetened, ½ cup	50
Apricots	
Canned, in syrup, ½ cup	110
Canned, in juice, ½ cup	43
Dried, 1 cup	390
Fresh, 2-3 medium	55
Banana, 1 medium	100
Blackberries, fresh, ½ cup	43
Blueberries	
Fresh, ½ cup	44
Frozen, 9 ounces	132
Cantaloupe, 5″ slice	30
Cherries	
Canned, in syrup, ½ cup	89
Fresh, ½ cup	40
Cranberries	
Fresh, 1 cup	46

Juice, 1 cup	165
Lo-cal, 1 cup	60
Sauce, 1 cup	405
Dates, fresh/dried, 1 cup	490
Figs	
Dried, 1 large	60
Fresh, 3 small	90
Fruit cocktail, ½ cup Fresh	100
Grapefruit, ½ medium	45
Juice, fresh, 1 cup	95
Grapes, ½ cup	33
Juice, 1 cup	135
Honeydew melon, 5″ slice	33
Lemon, 1 medium	20
Juice, 1 tablespoon	4
Lemonade, frozen, 1 cup	110
Mandarin oranges, 4 ounces	70
Maraschino cherry, 1	10
Nectarines, fresh, 2 medium	64
Orange, 1 medium	73
Juice, fresh, 1 cup	115
Frozen, 1 cup	120
Peaches	
2 halves, in syrup	90
Fresh, 1 medium	35
Pears	
2 halves, in syrup	90
Fresh, 1 medium	100
Pineapple	
Canned, ½ cup, in syrup	98
Fresh, ½ cup	38
Juice, 1 cup, unsweetened	135
Plums, 1 fresh	25
Pomegranate, 1 medium, fresh	63
Prunes, ½ cup, dried	148
Juice, 1 cup	200
Raisins, 1 cup	480
Raspberrries, fresh, 1 cup	50
Rhubarb, fresh, 1 cup	16
Strawberries, fresh, ½ cup	28
Frozen, sweetened, ½ cup	140

Tangerine, fresh, 1 medium	40
Watermelon, 4″ slice	115

VEGETABLES	CALORIES
Asparagus	
Canned, ½ cup	21
Fresh, ½ cup	15
Avocado, ½	185
Beans	
Baked, ½ cup	160
Green, ½ cup	15
Lima, ½ cup	130
Kidney, ½ cup	115
Beets, ½ cup	27
Broccoli, ½ cup	20
Brussels sprouts, ½ cup	28
Cabbage	
Cooked, ½ cup	20
Raw, 1 cup	20
Carrots	
Cooked, ½ cup	20
Raw, 1-2 large	42
Cauliflower	
Cooked, ½ cup	10
Raw, 1 cup	27
Celery, 2 stalks, raw	10
Coleslaw, ½ cup	58
Corn	
Canned, kernel, ½ cup	85
Fresh, 1 ear	70
Cucumber, 1 cup	5
Eggplant, cooked, ½ cup	19
Endive, raw, 1 head (20 leaves)	20
Lettuce, ½ head, iceberg	30
Mushrooms, canned, ½ cup	17
Olives, green, 4 medium	15
Onion	
Cooked, ½ cup	30
Raw, chopped, 2 tablespoons	10
Parsnips, ½ cup	50

Peas, ½ cup	58
Pepper, 1 medium	10
Pickles	
Dill, 1 large	15
Sweet, 1 large	45
Popcorn	
Plain, 1 cup	25
With oil, salt, 1 cup	45
Potatoes	
Baked, 1 medium	90
Boiled, 1 medium	80
French fries, 10-15	150
Fried, ½ cup	225
Mashed, ½ cup	63
Potato Chips, 10-12	120
Sweet Potatoes	
Baked, 1 medium	155
Candied, 1 medium	295
Potato salad, ½ cup	99
Pumpkin, 1 cup	75
Radishes, 4 medium	7
Romaine, 4 ounces	25
Rutabaga, ½ cup	35
Sauerkraut, ½ cup	20
Spinach, ½ cup	23
Squash, ½ cup	
Summer	15
Winter	65
Tomato, 1 medium	35
Paste, 3½ ounces	82
Juice, 1 cup	40
Turnip, ½ cup	20

MEATS/POULTRY	CALORIES
Bacon, 2 slices	90
Canadian bacon, 3 slices	195
Beef	
Corned, 3 ounces	185
Hamburger, 3-ounce patty	185
Liver, fried, 2 ounces	130
Pot roast, 2½ ounces	140

Rib roast, 2½ ounces	140
Round steak, 3 ounces	220
Sirloin steak, 3 ounces	330
Chop suey, 3½ ounces	120
Chicken	
Broiled, 3½ ounces	175
Fried, 3½ ounces	220
A la king, 3½ ounces	190
Chow mein, 3½ ounces	100
Pie, 4½-inch piece	535
Frankfurter, 1	140
Ham, 3½ ounces	220
Lamb	
Loin chop, 3½ ounces	223
Rib chop, 3½ ounces	290
Leg roast, 3½ ounces	195
Lunch meat	
Bologna, 1 slice	85
Boiled ham, 1 ounce	70
Salami, 1 slice	130
Meat loaf, beef & pork, 1 slice	265
Pork	
Pork chop, 3½ ounces	250
Sausage, 3½ ounces	420
Roast, 3½ ounces	240
Turkey, 3 slices	200
Veal	
Cutlet, 3½ ounces	200
Loin chop, 3 ½ ounces	200
Roast, 3½ ounces	175

FISH	CALORIES
Bass, baked, 3 ounces	215
Clam chowder, 8 ounce serving	
Manhattan, 1 serving	150
New England, 1 serving	260
Crab	
meat, ½ cup	85
Imperial, 1 serving	240
Fishstick, breaded, 1	40
Haddock, fried, 3 ounces	140

Halibut, broiled, 3 ounces	155
Perch, fried, 3 ounces	195
Salmon, broiled, 3 ounces	150
Pink, canned, ½ cup	185
Tuna	
in oil, ½ cup	160
in water, ½ cup	145
casserole, 1 serving	280
salad, 1 serving	170
Lobster	
½ cup	75
Thermidor, 1 serving	405
Mussels, 3½ ounces	95
Oysters	
on the half shell, 5-10 medium	80
stew, 1 cup	200
Scallops, 3½ ounces	112
Shrimp	
Broiled, 3 ounces	100
Fried, 3 ounces	190

DAIRY PRODUCTS	CALORIES
Butter, 1 tablespoon	100
Cheese	
Blue, 1 ounce	100
Cheddar, 1 ounce	120
Cottage, 1 cup	
Cream-style	240
Low fat	190
Cream cheese, 1 ounce	105
Neufchatel, 1 ounce	75
Parmesan, 1 tablespoon	20
Processed, 1 ounce	105
Swiss, 1 ounce	105
Cream	
Light, 1 tablespoon	30
Half-and-half, 1 tablespoon	20
Heavy, 1 tablespoon	55
Whipped, unsweetened, 1 tablespoon	30

199

Eggs
    Fried, 1   100
    Hard, soft, poached, 1   80
    Scrambled, 1   110
    White   15
    Yolk   60
Ice cream, 10% fat, ½ cup   130
Ice Milk, ½ cup   100
Margarine, 1 tablespoon   100
Milk
    Buttermijk, 1 cup   90
    Condensed, sweetened, ½ cup   500
    Evaporated, skim, ½ cup   85
    Evaporated, whole, ½ cup   170
    Skim, 1 cup   80
    Low fat, 2%, 1 cup   145
    Whole, 1 cup   160
Sour cream, ½ cup   240
    Low-cal, ½ cup   145
Yogurt
    Fruit, ½ cup   140
    Plain, low fat, ½ cup   65
    Plain, whole milk, ½ cup   75

BAKED PRODUCTS/SWEETS   CALORIES

Bread
    Biscuits, 1   145
    Corn, 1 square   95
    French, 1 slice   60
    Rye, 1 slice   60
    White, 1 slice   65
    Whole wheat, 1 slice   60

Cake
    Angel food, 1 slice   140
    Apple strudel, 1 slice   211
    Devil's food, 1 slice with
        chocolate frosting   600
    Fruit cake, 1 slice   155
    Gingerbread, 1 slice   180
    Pound cake, 1 slice   145

| Sponge cake, 1 slice | 200 |
| Yellow, 1 slice with chocolate frosting | 360 |

Cookies

Brownie, 1 piece	100
Chocolate chip, 1	50
Fig Newton, 1	50
Gingersnap, 1	30
Macaroon, 1	80
Sugar, 1	90
Vanilla wafer, 3	50

Crackers

Graham, 1	30
Saltine, 2	38
Soda, 2	50

Doughnut

Cake-type, 1	125
Yeast-type, 1	125
Jelly doughnut, 1	230
Honey, 1 tablespoon	65
Jam, 1 tablespoon	55
Maple syrup, 1 tablespoon	50
Marshmallow, 1	30

Muffins

| Blueberry, 1 | 120 |
| Corn, 1 | 150 |

Pancake

| Buckwheat, 1 | 55 |
| Plain, 1 | 60 |

Pie, 1 slice

Apple	400
Boston cream	200
Cherry	400
Lemon meringue	350
Mince	450
Pecan	570
Pumpkin	320

Pudding, ½ cup

Butterscotch	200
Chocolate	220
Tapioca	110
Vanilla	150

Rolls, hamburger
Sugar 90
    Brown, 1 tablespoon 50
    Granulated, 1 tablespoon 45
    Powdered, 1 tablespoon 30
Waffle, 1 200

CEREALS	CALORIES
Bran flakes, ¾ cup	100
Cream of Wheat, ¾ cup	96
Corn flakes, ¾ cup	70
Puffed oats, ¾ cup	80
Puffed rice, ¾ cup	40
Shredded wheat, ¾ cup	90
Soups, 1 cup	
Bouillon	30
Chicken noodle	70
Cream of mushroom, made with milk	200
Tomato, made with milk	170
Vegetable beef	80
Sandwiches	
Bacon, lettuce, tomato	280
Chicken salad	250
Egg salad	280
Boiled ham	280
Peanut butter	330
Tuna salad	275

INDEX

203

208